ALIGN YOUR HEALTH

Discover the essentials
to living a fulfilled,
healthy life.

DR. B.J. HARDICK

Illustration on page 37 © Dr. Ashly Ochsner

Photography on pages 233, 277, 275, 293, and 299 © Alieska Robles (alieskarobles.com)

The author extends special thanks to the numerous recipe contributors, photographers, and collaborators over the years and highest gratitude to Kimberly Roberto, co-author of *Maximized Living Nutrition Plans* (2009) and to Lin Hardick.

$25.00
ISBN 978-1-933936-93-2
52500>

9 781933 936932

I've been asked to endorse hundreds of books and authors. Perhaps every couple of years, I feel strongly enough about what's being written to do so. Dr. Hardick's book has stimulated me to step forward for two reasons.

First, we are suffering a health care crisis—not because of money, but because of intent and philosophy. We must end the thinking that health is the absence of disease. That's like believing the end of divorce would create healthy relationships. Dr. Hardick takes this philosophical battle head-on.

Second, you are not just reading Dr. Hardick's ideas and opinions; you are reading his life. He lives the principles in this book. He is a man of integrity and passion and a living example that health—in all its aspects—is founded on the powerful idea that we must first start with a respect for the intelligence of life and the understanding that health flows from from the inside out.

This book is a significant contribution to this growing body of knowledge that can change our lives, our health care system, and our world.

Dr. Guy Riekeman
Chancellor, Life University

Table of Contents

Table of Contents

Foreword

Our healthcare crisis has hit epidemic proportions. Chief among our problems is what I call diabesity, the spectrum of pre-diabetes to full-blown Type 2 diabetes, which now affects one out of two Americans and one in four children.

America's diabesity epidemic has reached staggering figures. The latest Centers for Disease Control and Prevention (CDC) statistics show 36.5 percent of Americans are obese and 86 million Americans have pre-diabetes (many of them don't know it!), paving the path for problems like Type 2 diabetes and heart disease.

Sadly, those statistics will only increase if people remain confused about what foods to eat or avoid. You know what I'm talking about: One day eggs are healthy; the next, experts say you should avoid them. Decades ago dietary fat got a bad rep; then scientists revealed certain fats could help you lose weight and feel better.

Lots of factors play into this confusion, including flawed reporting and biased studies. The $1 trillion food industry certainly does, with its "healthy" options like low-fat, high-fiber, whole-grain, and gluten-free, which are usually the opposite of healthy.

As a Functional Medicine doctor, I can see light within the darkness. Even amidst this confusion, I believe people are becoming more empowered to transform their health.

We now know that sugar, not dietary fat, is the real villain for diabesity. We're voting with our wallets by avoiding Frankenfoods for real, fresh, whole, organic foods. Grass-fed beef and wild-caught fish are in demand at many grocery stores.

More people are also becoming fed up with conventional medical advice that keeps them over-medicated yet undernourished. Rather than take a pill for a problem, they want to know what causes that problem and make deep-seated changes to heal it.

The foundation of that approach is Functional Medicine, which identifies and addresses the root causes of disease. Functional Medicine views the body as one integrated system, not a collection of independent organs divided up by medical specialties. It treats the whole system, not just the symptoms.

It's easy to think your biology is a lottery. Maybe you got the fat gene or a diabetes gene. Your parents are overweight, your grandparents were overweight, and diabetes runs in your family. There's not much you can do about it.

Functional Medicine says that yes, there is plenty you can do about it, even if your genetics tell you that you're overweight or prone to certain diseases. What you eat and how you live can activate your slim, healthy genes and silence your fat, sick genes.

Many present-day medical practitioners are bringing these principles into their practice because they work. They've seen how Functional Medicine empowers people to live healthier, happier lives without medications and other invasive procedures. Eastern medicine philosophers and chiropractors have espoused these principles as long as they've been around.

Dr. B.J. Hardick, a Canadian-based but world-renowned chiropractor, doesn't use the term Functional Medicine much in Align Your Health. However, his approach aligns perfectly with this philosophy.

The foundation to cultivating and maintaining vibrant health begins and ends with what you eat. Food is powerful medicine, and you can positively impact your health beginning with your very next meal.

But that's only one piece of the puzzle. Losing weight, reducing disease risk, and feeling better also require things like exercise, minimizing toxin exposure, and chiropractic principles like taking good care of your body structure.

Knowledge is power, and the right mindset helps you put these principles into action and sustain them over the long term. Throughout this book, Dr. Hardick provides powerful strategies to stay grounded, focused, optimistic, and resilient no matter what life throws your way.

Switching to real food, optimizing your nutrient status, and lowering your load of environmental toxins are among the powerful tools you'll learn about within these pages to help you reprogram your genes and optimize your health.

Altogether, the powerful and simple-to-implement practices in Align Your Health become potent medicine you can never replicate in a pill. This is powerful information you're holding in your hands, and it has the potential to change your life... One forkful, one simple action at a time.

Wishing you health and happiness,

— **Mark Hyman, MD**

Part One

Principles of Health

Chapter 1

Modern Health in Disarray

Chapter 2

Shifting Perspectives

CHAPTER 1

Modern Health in Disarray

By all surface measurements, this era should be the healthiest on record. Our access to information is through the roof. Most of us know the location of the nearest Whole Foods. Gyms, trainers, and fitness experts are, for many of us, our best friends—no longer just an annual resolution. Nutrition and food safety documentaries go viral, and we collectively follow every thought that our favorite wellness experts share in our social media feeds. We are learning more, attempting more, and seem to be taking care of our bodies more than ever before.

But are we actually taking care of ourselves? Chronic diseases are among the most preventable and prevalent health concerns in the country, yet the CDC estimates that 80 percent of all adults in the U.S. don't meet basic exercise recommendations, and 40 percent don't eat fruit or vegetables every day—not even once a day! (CDC, 2017) At the same time, healthcare costs in the U.S. have risen again, now up to $3.2 trillion annually, more than any other country in the world, with a full ten percent of those costs going to prescription drugs. (CDC, 2015) While the bulk of these expenses are attributed to cardiovascular diseases, diabetes, obesity, and other highly preventable concerns, pharmaceuticals are sold en masse as the solution. (Kanavos, et al, 2013) And people are wondering— *are* they even a solution?

What modern health has accomplished in minimizing infectious disease, it has lacked in the pursuit of health itself. We're reactively managing our disease instead of proactively controlling our health. We have lost sight of what it means to thrive: to wake with energy, fill our bodies with nutritious food, and enjoy life alongside friends and family. On some level, we're all looking for that in our lives; none of us wants to be sick, tired, and chained to prescriptions. Yet far too many of us— the majority, these stats seem to indicate—have accepted this new normal as unavoidable.

Hidden in Plain Sight

Visible illness typically gets more attention than chronic, hidden unhealth. A prime example of this sort of misdirection is America's ongoing war on obesity.

In the last several decades, the Western world has attempted to address the obesity epidemic in some rather counter-productive ways. You can now find more than 15,000 low-fat products on supermarket shelves—more than anywhere else in the world—as a direct reflection of our obsession with cutting dietary fat to lose body fat.

This approach has been ineffective in improving overall wellbeing, however; not only is obesity on the rise, but the focus on weight as a marker of health tends to cause caregivers to overlook dietary and hormonal imbalances that lead to inflammation and heart disease. Dr. Sylvan Lee Weinburg, the former president of the American College of Cardiology, wrote (Weinberg, 2004):

> *"The low-fat, high-carbohydrate diet... may well have played an unintended role in the current epidemics of obesity, type 2 diabetes, and metabolic syndromes. This diet can no longer be defended by appeal to the authority of prestigious medical organizations."*

To replace the lower fat content, carb intake has jumped, which we know to contribute to blood sugar and insulin issues, cancer, and obesity itself (as well as our most prevalent chronic, invisible plague: heart disease). Although doctors often endorse a diet low in fat, saturated fat, and cholesterol intake, there is little evidence to support it—much more on that in later chapters.

Despite our society's collective efforts, mortality rates from coronary heart disease, cancer, and diabetes have only increased over time. (Ford and Capewell, 2007)

Something isn't adding up.

Today, we're more aware that we're unhealthy and that conventional wisdom hasn't worked. But back when I wrote *Maximized Living Nutrition Plans* in 2009,

I found I almost had to prove to people that the North American continent was facing problems. Then, it was an uphill battle convincing readers that our solutions had withstood the test of time—and worked. But, today, the question isn't whether we need to change, but what to change first, and how.

No doubt, the awakening we've seen in the last five to ten years has driven people toward the opposite of convention—Paleo, or high-fat and protein diets—in droves. We know more now about healthy fats than we ever did in decades previous. Olive oil, avocados, nuts, seeds, and naturally-raised animal protein carry nutrients that our bodies need for healthy functions. And when we acknowledge that high-carb, low-fat diets have damaged our bodies, the natural tendency is to shift toward the opposite direction.

Carbohydrates, however, are an energy-producing food and necessary for the body to function optimally. Any diet that completely eliminates carbs is simply throwing the baby (fiber, energy, and micronutrients) out with the bathwater (refined sugars, fake foods, and high-glycemic carbs). What's more, artificial sweeteners have been marketed to this segment of the population, promising low-calorie, sugar-free versions of the things one might crave on a restrictive diet in a chemical-laden package.

We're still not there.

The marketing is effective. A simple trip to the grocery store can be overwhelming. The mixed messages we've been fed stack up to create difficult decisions. One survey of moms asked what they prioritize when they shop, and the results reflected the conflicting online advice that busy parents tend to rely on. (Womensforums.com, 2014) *Protein is good, so I must need something high-protein.* (79 percent of moms reached for high protein.) *This label says low-fat or low-calorie, so it should help my weight concerns.* (Nearly 70 percent for both.)

Labels must be read closely and carefully, and you've got to know what you're looking for. Most people still don't know what they need when they walk through the supermarket door, so they walk out with hidden, toxic ingredients and a completely imbalanced cart.

By no means do I want to add to the noise here by giving you more rules or contradictions. Quite the opposite. I want to help you learn to cut through the noise to be empowered to make healthy decisions for you and your family.

A Time for Everything

Western society has its dietary and lifestyle standards, but when illness is detected, quick remedies are far too often sought out as the answer. Whether it's medications or natural remedies, people want their fixes fast. Physician friends and colleagues of mine who work in the both the conventional medical system and in the broader field of natural health know and see this—and most wish the system today allowed for something better. While many interventions are required to save peoples' lives when in a state of emergency or crisis, our Western practices have driven many of us to expect health to come from a bottle. This is today's difficult dilemma. I believe that people inherently know that remedies and quick fixes aren't their saviour or long-term solutions—but they're all-too-easy to apply.

But true healing comes from within—not from outside-in.

Growing up, my own family doctor was my next door neighbor. He and my many other colleagues in medicine would say to this day that prescriptions alone do not *make* a person well. But, many may help to create conditions that enable someone to live better within the context of their disease. Ultimately, the doctor-patient relationship is one to be respected and preserved. Very specifically, any prescription or recommendation for medication should be evaluated on a case-by-case basis as an MD and patient work together to determine what's best for them.

Although you'll read success stories in this book from individuals who have been able to come off medications, no one can promise your complete recovery from a medication-regulated condition. There's simply no way to fulfill that promise. But, that's not the point—we're looking for wellness of the body and mind, not to usurp a doctor-patient relationship.

Unfortunately, the spiral of the western lifestyle, which for most people, includes an increasing number of prescriptions every year, often leads to more pills to fix more side effects and concurrent problems. Without addressing the cause, you're left spending more and feeling worse with no end in sight.

Our goal is to see you healthy, independent of that system. The premise is simple: if we can take better care of ourselves, we'll need fewer visits to the doctor. Patients are happier. (Doctors are happier, too—they can dedicate their years of schooling to advanced and complicated cases and medical emergencies, not to the common cold and lifestyle-preventable damage.) When you make those changes, your doctor will thank you for it—and your body's experience of good health will thank you, too.

The MaxLiving™ Story

What is the ultimate blind spot in restrictive diets and prescription-dependence? *There's no magic bullet.* You cannot eliminate a food group, create a new product, or take a simple supplement that will create a healthy lifestyle all in itself.

For all of the attempts to cut fat or lower carbs to lose weight, North Americans remain stressed, sedentary, and sleepless. Inflammatory illnesses and chronic pain plague us. Our minds and focus are in disarray. We struggle with migraines and back pain, yet we hunch over our desks, tip our necks to scroll through our phones, and remain slouched in seats and couches for most of the day. To truly overcome chronic illness, we need to make changes in our bodies, movements, habits, and minds.

This information is not new to chiropractors. Classically, a chiropractor's goal is to eliminate interference that keeps the body from achieving wellness. For generations, chiropractors have watched their patients' lives improve with their alignment, never mind the lifestyle changes and attention to nutrition.

But at the turn of the millennium, in a world that was getting sicker and sicker, my colleagues and I took a serious look at what our own patients, friends and family members were doing in order to thrive. Ultimately, it came down to use a group of principles I learned courtesy of a program established as the 5 Essentials™ which was developed by Maximized Living. Following the principles of this program consistently led to not only healthier lives, but a reversal of the negative outcomes individuals had already endured. In the chapters ahead, it is my intention to communicate the principles underlying the 5 Essentials approach to you and to health seekers and advocates beyond the network of MaxLiving™ practitioners and their patients.

I would point out that, in twenty years, although much has changed in the world of natural health, this model of wellness remains anchored in the principles underlying the 5 Essentials program. Practices and applications may have refined, but principles have not.

5 Essentials™

This simple and effective approach to health care focuses on chiropractic care, simple and clean nutrition, a clear mindset, oxygen and exercise, and minimizing toxin exposure. Each of the essentials can become a focus individually or in combination, and each will bring you closer to whole-body health.

Chiropractic in Practice and in Principle

All too often, chiropractic care is relegated to pain-control. Patients view the chiropractor as another facet of western health care, only there to mitigate symptoms as they arise. Although this has become the accepted standard of chiropractic care—it's far from the traditional principles behind the profession.

The chiropractic philosophy of health is centered on the spine. And why not? Your spine runs through the center of your body, connecting all systems, every organ, and ultimately each cell to one another. An optimal nerve expression allows each component of your body to work in concert with the others. The core principle of traditional chiropractic care is to keep the spine and nervous system free of structural interferences that everyday stressors create. Prioritizing spinal alignment is an important first step toward unlocking your body's natural potential for health and healing.

Nutrition

The food we eat affects weight, disease prevention, mental and emotional health, and overall wellbeing. And when chiropractors and other holistic health providers speak of cellular regeneration, they recognize that cells do not regenerate from thin air but from the molecules available to the body from the food we eat.

Every process in the body is fueled in some way by food, for better or for worse. Imbalanced diets not only leave you feeling weighed down and sluggish, but they leave you susceptible to disease, as well.

Rather than advocating a one-size-fits-all nutritional guide, the MaxLiving philosophy acknowledges that we are all different. It accepts that numbers are subjective and that a healthy body composition is more important than mere weight loss. We emphasize that increased energy, reduced inflammation, and improved immunity and resilience are some of the most important effects of a healthy diet. To accomplish this, we seek to empower you to create your own nutritional blueprint that helps you both understand and solve your body's unique needs.

Mindset

Underlying physical change is a mindset of success. How many times have you found yourself determined to pursue a goal—change your diet, begin an exercise routine, start a new habit—only to run into burnout and "cheats" after a short time? Without a renewed, refocused mindset free of conflicting societal messages, it can be difficult (or impossible!) to commit to the 5 Essentials program.

A mindset shift can become a goal for change in itself, as well. Time management, sleep prioritization, and stress reduction support healthy brain and body function. With mental, emotional, and physical health in focus, you can better pursue the essential actions that lead to holistic health.

Oxygen & Exercise

Exercise is a universal recommendation for better health, but in this book, we'll explore a unique approach to exercise that digs deeper than the traditional surface—one that is not only grounded in science, but easy to apply in life. An effective exercise routine should be practical in the face of time constraints and busy lifestyles. It should bring more oxygen into the body, to feed both body and mind. It should build lean muscle and improve performance.

Not just exercise, but the right *kind* of exercise affects your hormone levels, immune system, body fat, mental health, and emotional stability. In other words: we don't want to see you pour any more precious time or unfulfilled hopes into yet another unsuccessful exercise program.

Minimize Toxins

MaxLiving philosophy acknowledges the body's ability to effectively and permanently remove toxins from cells. The body's detoxification system is elegant and thorough when it functions optimally. But we place significant stressors on this system at every turn, from personal care items, interactions with foods, air quality in our own home, and—there's no way to put this nicely—quite often the medications we take to help us. Combined with pollution and aromatics from home cleaning products and perfumes, this onslaught is enough to inhibit optimal functions in our body, threatening health and longevity. And this science is clear— you'll read about it later.

When we minimize toxin exposure, the body gets a chance to breathe a bit easier (literally and figuratively), detoxify more efficiently, and perform on a higher level.

Simple, Profound Changes

The world wants answers to its compounding, confounding health questions. How can we overcome chronic illness? Why is obesity rampant? What causes us to lose energy and *joie de vivre*? The more we try to solve these problems, the worse we seem to make things for ourselves.

There may not be a single, simple answer to unlock the mysteries of wellness. There won't be a one-size-fits-all plan that fits everyone. But we believe there are common factors and shared principles that drive us toward health. In my experience as an individual pursuing personal health—and as a Doctor of Chiropractic observing thousands of patients doing the same—I can confidently say that these shared principles are captured in the 5 Essentials. We can make simple yet profound changes that will eventually change our lives. And, by the time you finish this book, you will have the knowledge, the power, and the tools available to align your health.

CHAPTER 2
Shifting Perspectives

More than ever before, our friends, neighbors, and family members want more out of life than to not be sick. We want to be well. We want to thrive. We want a philosophy of health that eliminates dis-ease, but from deeper than conventional medicine can reach.

And while I don't believe one has to be religious to embrace a holistic philosophy of health, there's a growing movement to embrace health inclusively from a spiritual, emotional, and physical place.

As far back as 1948, the **World Health Organization** defined health as "a state of complete physical, mental, and social well-being—and not merely the absence of disease or infirmity." (WHO, 2017) Pope John Paul II reinforced this sentiment when he elaborated, "Health is a dynamic tension towards physical, mental, social and spiritual harmony, and not only the absence of illness."(Fos, 2011)

From the Roman spas to the rise of Christianity, healthcare has always been enmeshed with philosophy. We see Hippocrates declaring "do no harm," and primary methods of healing shifting with the philosophical bent of each given era. In the modern era, unfortunately, mainstream healthcare has been divorced from philosophy. The historical philosophy of health is about connecting with people as a whole being, allowing them to retain their autonomy, and maintaining access to care for every single person.

Weigh that legacy of medicine and healing with our modern focus on the absence of disease, and the contrast is stark. Now, we have payments, insurance, and healthcare as a privilege rather than a right, and authority rather than autonomy. (NCBI, 2017)

Whether or not you have identified it yet, we all carry our own philosophy of health. It's acted out in the way we think about our bodies and lives, the way we eat, the habits we form, and the practitioners we frequent. Many of us were raised with a philosophy that we may grow out of with time and critical thought. Perhaps you are here because you have grown weary of the results you've had to live with as a result of adhering to these old ideas.

A Philosophy of Wellness

We simply believe that the body is designed to be healthy. It is a philosophy of innate wellness, in which we can do nothing to cause healing or health of our own volition. Stick with me: this is not a message of helplessness. Instead, our bodies are *intended* to be healthy, and that force of innate strength—the same invisible force that creates life and ends it—drives us constantly toward wellness.

The holistic and chiropractic view of health is that interference with this natural function is what causes disease. More accurately, *dis-ease*. Even when an illness is not diagnosed, anything that sets our bodies, minds, spirits, and emotions on edge is dis-ease and, to the MaxLiving philosophy of health, an effect of interference.

This can also be described as or associated with the philosophy of vitalism, in contrast with the conventional or more mainstream philosophy of health, which is rooted in mechanism.

Mechanism is allopathic, seeking to treat and repair. It views the body as a collection of matter: the protons, neurons, and electrons. The tissues and organs and parts. Mechanism can be put under a microscope to measure and quantify visible changes.

Vitalism, on the other hand, is less tangible. It is concerned with the unseen energies that connect the cells of one's being. It recognizes that some things won't show up under a microscope. That humans are unique, even though our mechanics are similar.

Mechanism looks at parts of the body; vitalism looks at the life in the body.

Mechanism studies populations; vitalism studies individuals.

Mechanism deals in matter; vitalism deals in life.

A chiropractic view of the world—and the MaxLiving philosophy of health—prioritizes this innate sense of wellness as the driving force behind all of our interactions. We are constantly looking for that sense, learning to listen closely to it, and removing any interference that may stand in the way.

This is not a new concept, by any stretch of the imagination. Philosophers have long discussed the importance of energy and the unseen. It is the *space between the notes of music* that Wayne Dyer so eloquently refers to. The idea that it is in the "space between our thoughts that everything is created." We see the philosophy of vitalism and importance of energy and individualism illustrated by researchers and experts like the conventionally-trained Drs. Deepak Chopra and Andrew Weil. It's a concept that emerged in the earliest forms of Eastern medicine and lasted through the generations to seep into the philosophies of top scientists today.

Not everyone will share the same philosophy of health; this we can all respect. What we must recognize is that your philosophy will determine your actions, guide your choices, and, ultimately, bring you confidence in making those decisions. It was Bernie Siegel, MD—as he examined cancer survivors while writing his best-selling book, *Love, Medicine and Miracles*—who identified a shining thread amongst survivors: faith, confidence, and belief in their doctors and in the treatments they were receiving. Yes, your philosophy does influence your actions—and your belief influences your outcomes. In a world full of options with respect to nutrition, never mind the broader field of health care choices, authors like Bruce Lipton, Ph.D. (*"The Biology of Belief"*), and countless others between him and Siegel, will tell you for certain: mindset matters. More on mindset at the conclusion of this book.

What's the philosophy shared by MaxLiving, traditional chiropractic, and vitalism? **Your body is driven for health and wholeness and will strive to achieve it, provided there is no interference.**

Throughout *Align Your Health*, we will relay as much information as we can, as thoroughly as we can, for you to apply it in any way that you can. But it is all based on a foundation that you are powerful beyond measure. You deserve and can achieve a life of vitality, free of interference in all of its forms.

In MaxLiving, we use this philosophical underpinning to build toward the practical, evidenced-backed principles taught in this book.

Sources of Interference

Interference can show up in countless ways, most of which are triggered by our own decisions and practices. Interference can happen suddenly, or for a short period of time. It can be chronic, building slowly and quietly, without notice. Most sources of interference can be grouped into one of three categories of stressors:

- Physical Stress
- Chemical Stress
- Emotional Stress

Physical Stress

Since we are in the mindset of a chiropractor-patient relationship at the moment, some physical stressors might seem obvious. Poor posture can place unnatural stress on parts of the spine, leading to soreness and pain that brings you in for an adjustment. After the adjustment, your back feels better and you move on with your life.

Sometimes, though, you notice the adjustment leads to other areas of your body feeling better or functioning better. This is not because of any particular skill on the chiropractor's part, but because the interference in the spinal column had been removed in the adjustment, freeing your body to address hidden problems with oxygenation, nervous system integrity, and nutrients. B.J. Palmer, D.C., the developer of the chiropractic profession, professed that every cell in the body needs access to these components! It was also in the Palmer tenets that interference blocks the integrity of the nervous system and, therefore, hinders health from a cellular level.

Other forms of physical stress might block oxygenation and nutrients. This can look like inadequate sleep, injuries, physically demanding work, a sedentary lifestyle, unreasonably strenuous exercise, poor breathing—more on these in chapter five. Any instance of the parts and pieces of your body being mistreated, misused, and maladjusted can become a physical stressor and interfere with innate processes that should lead to health.

Chemical Stress

Again, let's look at our first most obvious example: interactions with toxins interfere with the body's original design. Though we are born with intricate detoxification pathways—the liver constantly cleaning blood, the excretory process, sweat and fluid balance—we can still become mired in the effects of toxins. Why? Because of interference within the environment.

The body is bombarded with toxins all day and night. Our homes, schools, and offices are built and cleaned with toxic materials, and we are closed up inside of them for hours on end. Our toiletries, clothes, and food bring an onslaught of toxins in small and large amounts at every turn. Our lungs, skin, and digestive tract stay on high alert, in constant response to the world around us. These are sources of interference that we'll take a close look at in chapter six.

A key facet of the westernized, mechanistic philosophy of health is that it attempts to heal with chemical adjustments to address symptoms of disease, where the MaxLiving philosophy expects healing to be driven by the innately-driven healing abilities of the body itself.

Though no one would deny the use of life-saving drugs once other options are exhausted, the side-effects that medications carry cannot be overlooked. In other words, medication can be a form of chemical interference, and there can be a price to pay for benefits gained. This is all the more reason to be an informed, active part of your journey toward innate health, always learning and weighing the risks and benefits of an intervention.

We should think critically not only about intervention, but also the philosophy behind it. Even many practitioners of natural health still hold a mechanistic philosophy, recommending interference in the form of vitamins and supplements or prescribed nutrition to *alter* biochemical processes in the body. However, I would consider a recommendation of vitamins and supplements to provide the body with nutrients it is missing as a result of modernization—a vitalistic recommendation. It's not trying to force change, but rather, allow the body to express *itself*.

Let me explain: Good foods are there to nourish our bodies. Supplements can provide nutrients where diet and lifestyle might come up short, so there certainly can be a place for those "natural remedies," even in a MaxLiving life, as we'll explore in chapter seven. Where the philosophies diverge, however, is when the food and supplements and products become *mechanisms* to force change.

Even when it's branded as natural—which, as a definition in itself can get sticky, since everything comes from the earth at some point—forcing an outcome from an external source can be a form of interference. If you're feeling weighed down with a stack of remedies and "natural" pills, consider the philosophy that might drive your natural care practitioner to recommend them. Consider whether this is the philosophy you'd prefer to align with.

Emotional Stress

Mental and emotional health is difficult to maintain, resolve, or even notice in many parts of the world. We move through life at such a rapid pace, practically worshiping the tangible results we gain from productivity and busyness. The same goes for health, as we've seen with massive campaigns against obesity or the vices without any care for what has created the emotional need to overeat or turn to a vice in the first place. In this way, "stress" as we understand it is an emotional stress.

The effects of emotional stress as interference can be measured in terms of hormonal shifts. We can point to fight or flight, cortisol, and the effects these imbalances have on the brain and body. As researchers learn more about the effects of stress, this is the language that they have developed to measure and quantify its effects.

From a MaxLiving perspective—not merely an attempt to remove and replace a broken piece—emotional stress can be completely intangible. We can use that language, as you'll see in chapter eight, but we don't need it. The deepest question of interference is this: what stands in between the physical body and the Innate Intelligence that runs it? What keeps us from aligning with the invisible, innate forces that keep our cells connected and vibrating from conception, until our very last breath?

From this philosophical standpoint, from a lifestyle that embraces the 5 Essentials, we don't look for interference or innate wellness to use them as tools. Instead, they are core functions of our being that we always seek to understand and facilitate. This is why mindset is one of the 5 Essentials.

Removing Interference

If we are bombarded with interference in so many different ways, then, how can we possibly begin to clear it all away to regain that innate health? The MaxLiving philosophy will not try to pretend that your answer will be the same as your spouse's or your neighbor's or mine. You've likely already picked up on this in your own observations. Why can one person drink soda regularly and not get ill, while another takes a sip and immediately feels the effects? Why are there so many different diet plans that seem to work or not work inexplicably? Why can two very different chiropractic adjustments lead to equally improved health?

One philosophy of health, mechanism, will muse about all of the potential factors and reasons that certain bodies react differently than others. The other, MaxLiving, says that the external actions matter—but it's the body's ability to respond and adapt to the environment that matters most. And because no two people are the same, we don't always know how a body will respond when interference is removed. From this perspective, the MaxLiving perspective on health is simply to identify interference, reduce it or remove it, and let the body harness its innate recuperative powers to heal on its own.

Simple Adjustments

Of the 5 Essentials, we prioritize core chiropractic care first. Why? It's often the simplest change you can make to remove interference. Recall that you can work on one essential or a combination, because any interference removed is better than none. When you routinely visit a chiropractor focused on removing interference, the adjustments are simple but can be profound. Often, when individuals receive a very specific, but not lengthy chiropractic adjustment, they may say, "That's it?" The answer is yes. As chiropractic pioneer Dr. Clarence Gonstead used to say with respect to correcting problems in the body, "Find it. Fix it. Leave it alone." The principle of identifying interference, removing interference, and then allowing the body to heal *itself* is at the core of classic chiropractic philosophy.

It was Dr. B.J. Palmer who said: *Medicine is the study of disease and what causes man to die. Chiropractic is the study of health and what causes man to live.*

Sometimes, an adjustment will remove interference that affects the body in surprising and exciting ways. You feel better, move better, and find seemingly unrelated health problems begin to alleviate. Other times, as the body awakens and establishes new patterns, you begin to feel for the very first time—you begin to realize just how badly you never knew you felt. From a mechanistic perspective, you might be inclined to wonder if you are feeling funky because you needed to do more or less before or after your adjustment. You could even be faced with this wonder when responding oddly to other positive changes in your life, such as eliminating sugar, gluten, or sleeping more—you name it. The difference, however, is that the MaxLiving philosophy has a profound respect for your body's Innate Intelligence—and sometimes, when you make positive changes, your body will first begin to wake up and even feel uncomfortable as the healing begins. Make the right changes—then trust in the process. **Never underestimate the power of the body to heal itself.**

A Lifestyle of Change

While chiropractic is often one's first step toward removing interference, it's not the last. When patients visit a chiropractor with issues varying from cancer to irritable bowel disease to headaches, or simply a lifestyle of stress, a chiropractor will start with an adjustment for the purpose of reducing interference in the body—but no chiropractor can predict exactly how one's body will respond.

Moving forward, it's up to each person to create a lifestyle of change that removes interference. You see, I believe it shouldn't be up to anyone else to tell you to remove or add "this or that." No. I ultimately wish for you to become free of interference, and therefore empowered to trust in your body's own Innate Intelligence. To understand what kinds of things cause interference, identify their effect on your own life, and hear your own body telling you what you need. I want you to become self-driven, self-aware, and ultimately, self-healing.

The actions themselves are secondary to the philosophy. Soda doesn't make you sick; interference does. Green juice doesn't make you well; your body's Innate Intelligence does. We see this philosophy shared in vitalism, eastern and Chinese medicine, and in chiropractic care pioneered by D.D. Palmer and B.J. Palmer. There is a broad understanding, outside of our conventional medicine in the Western world, that respects the body's knowledge of what it wants and needs to be well. This understanding acknowledges that a Universal Intelligence—which some call God, and others call Mother Nature—placed this desire and ability in our bodies.

While there are some lessons you can learn in a lab, there are some lessons you learn in life. There are many understandings you come to by listening closely to your body and giving it what it needs.

Counter-Philosophy: Mechanism

As you move through this book and begin to recognize points of interference in your own life, don't forget to check in with your body as well. The actions alone, apart from the philosophy that drives them, will not be as powerfully effective. As an example, adding green juice into your diet or starting chiropractic care, without committing to a lifestyle that removes interference, will only do so much. Focusing exclusively on specific actions would be the Westernized approach—in an attempt to treat, to remedy, to force an outcome—and this is driven by a philosophy of mechanism.

But that's not what we are talking about in this book or pursuing as part of the 5 Essentials. Mechanism runs directly counter to the MaxLiving philosophy and the vitalistic worldview. It attributes the action, or the supplement, or the food, or the drug, or the habit for doing the healing. A MaxLiving life pursues the 5 Essentials while recognizing that there is an inborn healing potential within the body, and that the body is driven towards a state of well-being. It recognizes that body is *self*-healing. It's our job, first, to remove the interference.

Align Your Philosophy

MaxLiving is not a replacement for medicine. But, for all of the assumptions the drug era is just beginning, it seems much more realistic that people are seeking transformations that the drug era has never been able to offer. People want something more substantial.

People are looking for a lifestyle of wellness, with drugs and surgery implemented only when necessary. They want a way to make that a reality in their own lives. Perhaps this drive comes from the whispers of Innate Intelligence itself.

When we look for one simple answer, we mix the complex foundational truths. The more mechanism learns, the more vitalism—the mystery of life—is confirmed. We draw from the wisdom and knowledge that science observes and apply it in practice alongside the philosophy that the body is much greater than the sum of its individual parts. When there is harmony in the body, an overall state of peace, and a lack of interference, there is health. Disconnects lead to chaos. This is our philosophy of health, and the beauty and empowerment of it is this: you get to decide whether you align with it.

Part Two

Practical Essentials

Chapter 3

Chiropractic at the Core

Chapter 4

Eat Well to Live Well

Chapter 5

Innate Movement

Chapter 6

Freeing the Body of Toxins

Chapter 7

Essential Supplementation

Chapter 8

Mindset for Life

CHAPTER 3

Chiropractic at the Core

Visiting a chiropractor is not an abnormal thing to do. Many health insurance providers cover the visit, and doctors will usually accept it as "complementary" or "alternative" (and may even prescribe the visit!). In these appointments, patients and clients come to chiropractors ready to fix their back pain, relieve their posture-related problems, and release pinched nerves. These are all good things! But it's only half the story. As a science, philosophy, and art, chiropractic principles sit at the core of the 5 Essentials.

When we begin to envision our lives as they could be and our health as it should be, the urge to change everything at once can be tempting. But bear this in mind: even though there are only 5 Essentials, we're going to cover a *lot* of ground in this book. Rather than becoming overwhelmed and giving up, starting with the simple addition of chiropractic care can be an easy first addition, with a big payoff.

Chiropractic is concerned with the nervous system—and the nervous system affects every part of your body and mind. The entire spinal cord is housed in and protected by the spinal column. Every pair of spinal nerves exits the spinal cord between two corresponding vertebral bones, above and below. The fundamental principle of chiropractic, since its inception, has always stated that any interference to the function of those nerves as a result of spinal misalignment or mechanics will cause dysfunction in the corresponding cells, organs, and systems of the body.

These points of impairment are called subluxations, and they can occur in specific segments of the spine or in full regions, such as the neck. Keeping them at bay will free your body to approach health even as you work to incorporate the other essentials into your life. And, a body that's functioning poorly on the inside is forever going to be limited in its response to good nutrition, exercise, optimal mindset, and detoxification from the outside.

Lifestyle isn't Enough

Unfortunately, the typical Western lifestyle is not supportive of good health. Fast-paced, work-driven schedules and consumption-driven habits have altered the ways our bodies and minds respond to the world around us. Our stress hormones are always turned on, creating long-term inflammation and limiting mental and emotional capabilities. Our digestive systems are maxed out as they attempt to thrive on the processed food products that we turn to during stressful days. Heart disease, diabetes, and cancers are rampant, not just in worst-case scenarios, but in the majority of adults.

In contrast with chiropractic, public health experts, conventional physicians, and wellness coaches often point to lifestyle changes first, asking their clients and patients to simply *do* better to feel better. *If only* you ate better foods. *If only* you exercised more. *If only* you resisted the tendency toward stress. If you could "only" make better choices, then your body would be happier and healthier.

Though not entirely wrong, this advice is incomplete. We can all point to at least one person in our lives who lives a healthy lifestyle and has still wound up sick—either acute illnesses or chronic. Sometimes, the attempt at a healthy lifestyle itself makes people sick, such as athletes who overtrain, for example. Other times, the illness seems inexplicable. "They did everything right," we say, "Of all the people to fall ill...is there no hope for the rest of us?"

The role of stress in illness lies at the heart of the chiropractic philosophy, but chiropractors look to see whether the stressors are within the body, instead of external. **Stressors are not only emotional and biochemical; they can be physical.**

That's where chiropractic comes in. Whatever interferes with the natural function of the body should be removed, first and foremost. This is such a simple step forward that anyone can make. It allows the body to work better without any difficult lifestyle changes. It's beneficial for everyone, regardless of habits or perceived health.

The First Essential

Chiropractors examine the spine for abnormalities that should be corrected—or, as we affirm in chiropractic, adjusted. These exams might involve x-rays, visual analysis, palpation checks or physical testing. Spinal abnormalities and areas of subluxation can include segmental or regional misalignments, improper movement, degenerative and pathological changes, and corresponding stressors on the central nervous system. According to the Association of Chiropractic Colleges, later adopted by the World Federation of Chiropractic: (WFC, 2001 and ACC, 2017)

"Chiropractic is concerned with the preservation and restoration of health, and focuses particular attention on the subluxation. A subluxation is a complex of functional and/or structural and/or pathological articular changes that compromise neural integrity and may influence organ system function and general health. A subluxation is evaluated, diagnosed, and managed through the use of chiropractic procedures based on the best available rational and empirical evidence."

This definition of the subluxation complex was affirmed by all Presidents and/or Deans of the sixteen chiropractic institutions in North America in 1996. With expanded research efforts over the past two decades, a consortium of six chiropractic schools plus three emerging institutions representing global efforts across the United States, Europe, Central America, China and New Zealand, known as *The Rubicon Group*, enhanced its definition of the chiropractic subluxation as:

"...a self-perpetuating, central segmental motor control problem that involves a joint, such as a vertebral motion segment, that is not moving appropriately, resulting in ongoing maladaptive neural plastic changes that interfere with the central nervous system's ability to self-regulate, self-organize, adapt, repair and heal."

Excuse the scientific terminology. In essence, the chiropractic institutions committed to the natural approach to health and well-being, excluding the practice of drugs and surgery, recognize one thing: **Structure influences function.**

Chiropractors look for what's wrong in the spinal alignment and fix it, based on the foundational understanding that the spine is the anchor of the body and at the center of health. While there are countless unique methods of chiropractic analysis and intervention—some performed by hand, others performed using tools and instruments —the chiropractic perspective is that simple.

When we refer to the nervous system, two components are included: the central nervous system and the peripheral nervous system. The central nervous system (CNS) runs along the spinal column and includes the brain and brain stem, while the peripheral nervous system (PNS) branches out into the organs and limbs. When you touch a hot stove, the PNS sends pain signals through the CNS to the brain, and the brain returns the message to pull your hand away. Another function of the PNS is its autonomic, or involuntary controls, including things like digestive control and cardiovascular function.

But it is the central nervous system itself that carries everything from movement, sensation, and thought processes from brain to body and back again. And this system is enclosed within and protected by the vertebrae of the spine.

All About the Spine

An adult spine is comprised of 24 vertebrae, extending between the skull and the pelvis. The vertebrae are grouped into categories: cervical, thoracic, lumbar, sacral, and coccygeal. The vertebrae themselves are interlocking bones, and they are separated by spinal discs that cushion and support them. Nestled within this interlocking, flexible column of bones lies the spinal cord, which connects directly to the brain.

In a normal, healthy spine, there are curves at each section. The seven cervical vertebrae should create a gentle inward curve at the base of your head. The twelve thoracic vertebrae move outward at the shoulders and back in toward the lumbar spine, where five more vertebrae create the gentle arch of the small of your back. Finally, the fused sacral vertebrae that create the sacrum and the fused coccygeal vertebrae of the tailbone curve back out as part of the buttocks.

Apart from housing the nervous system, the spinal column helps to anchor muscles throughout the body. Good posture, muscle strength, and spinal health are all interconnected. Weakness across the upper back will hunch shoulders beyond the normal rounding of the thoracic spine. Exaggerating the lower lumbar curve in the small of your back—as is often the case during pregnancy—can strain the normal tension of muscles in the abdomen and lead to diastasis recti or abdominal wall separation. Similarly, consider that the sacrum and tailbone anchor the pelvic floor and bladder, and that weak posture and balance can stress everything that's housed within the pelvic region.

So we can see that, even before a chiropractor looks for subluxation—the slips, misalignment, pinched nerves, pain, and asymptomatic quirks—these can have major, whole-body implications on spine health. And that's just a little bit of what's related to posture!

Now, still picturing the spine as an anchor to the whole body, take the nervous system into consideration. The nerves that communicate and connect with every limb, system, organ, and area of the body are bundled together and protected within the vertebral column. When spinal health is ideal, a perfect column is formed for the spinal cord to run unimpeded to the brain. Every natural bend of the spine is intended and relates to the protection of these nerves.

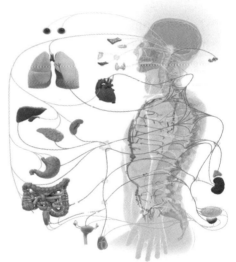

It becomes clear, then, that shifts in vertebral alignment can not only alter posture, lead to muscular discomfort, and, in worse cases, bone-on-bone pain, but can extend throughout the body with extensive repercussions.

Spinal Abnormalities

With the spine at the literal center of our bodies and health, keeping it protected and aligned becomes an obvious priority. But even the healthiest lifestyle can create abnormalities in the spine. Why? Because our world is not built for a healthy spine, and it takes careful intentionality to take care of this hidden but vital piece of wellness.

From the very beginning of our lives—the shifting and sometimes trauma of birth can lead to subluxation or abnormalities in the vertebral column. A chiropractor, then, is as much a partner for life as a physician, optimizing your health through life's everyday stresses as well as in case of major damage.

Spinal Trauma

The most obvious type of spinal abnormality comes with direct trauma. Direct or indirect spinal trauma usually lead to back and neck pain, which has become the most studied, well-accepted reason for chiropractic adjustments.

Spinal trauma can refer to the most obvious concerns: car accidents, falls, and sports injuries. Any time a traumatic external force affects the body, the spine will take the impact. Part of the design of the vertebrae—interlocking but flexible, cushioned at all intersections—is to be able to withstand most forces. Jumping, falling, running, and even sitting are all stressors on the spine that have to be mitigated in some way.

A healthy spine can support your body weight and the stressors of daily life. But the more your body and spine fall into disrepair, the less trauma and stress it can take. In that scenario, prolonged time in a desk chair or couch, carrying around excess body weight, and everyday occurrences can add up to spinal trauma. You might notice it as regular discomfort, or it might be invisible until you reach for something in the attic and "throw your back out."

Posture

The average Western lifestyle—even among the most health-conscious—is terrible for posture. From our shoes to our chairs to our limited walking, our world is not set up for good alignment. It takes a conscious effort to keep the spine and muscles controlled and in line with good posture.

Consider this: When you stand up, if you were to hang a string from the top of your head to the ground, how would your body align with it? Would your ears be over your shoulders or pressed forward? Do your shoulders square above your hips or have they slumped? What does the line between your shoulders look like? Is there a slight bend at your lower back, or has it pulled into a dramatic curve as your stomach muscles have given way? Are your knees locked and rigid, overworking to compensate?

What about this: if you were to sit on the floor, could you get up unassisted? Could you do it without rolling over onto your knees?

Incidentally, our standing posture is probably damaged the most by our sitting postures. In a vicious cycle of negative feedback, the soft chairs and couches that seem to relieve an aching back curve the body into an unnatural position. Without proper support of the sitz-bones and lower back, the upper back hunches. Eventually, the muscle tone that holds our bodies in alignment breaks down, and the correct posture becomes uncomfortable. Then we want to relax into a soft chair, and so the cycle continues.

Stress

Stress is connected with all sorts of health concerns, from heart disease to chronic pain and headaches. Incidentally—and not at all a coincidence—so are spinal abnormalities. We could think of them as a chicken and egg situation: which came first, the abnormality or the stress? But that's a more linear view of health than what we hope to achieve.

Instead, we approach wellness as something that's interconnected. Poor spinal health can certainly interfere with the function of the heart and pathways of inflammation. Adjustments can relieve headaches, among many other things. And stress—though it plays it own role in a variety of ailments and discomfort—can also affect spinal health. (Bryans, et al, 2011)

How? When we become stressed, we hold our bodies differently. We pull our shoulders taut. We hunch. We keep our muscles tensed. Each of these unconscious movements pulls the natural tension in our bodies out of sorts and, with the muscles anchored on the spine, pull the spine out of alignment. What's more, stress starts a pro-inflammatory response in the body that can affect the discs, ligaments, and tendons around the spine. Again, leading to pain and creating spinal abnormalities.

Repeating Patterns

Spine health is often left out of sight, out of mind, but the small things in life add up. Long before pain shows up, basic lifestyle habits and oversights can wreak cumulative havoc on the spine. The bed in which you sleep, the pillows you use, and the sleep habits you foster all contribute to alignment and inflammation that can cause spinal abnormalities. In the rush of the morning, exercise is often replaced with sitting and more sitting. Rushing through breakfast, carpooling to work, driving kids to school, sitting in a desk—our lives are fast-paced mentally and sedentary physically.

Sometimes, when we are able to prioritize exercise, the things we think are helping are actually doing more damage. When you do make time to exercise, how careful are you in your movements? Are you aware of form when you strength train or hop on the treadmill?

What shoes are you wearing, from work to errands to eveningwear? The shoes built for style are rarely built for the health of the spine. Walking in flip flops, dress shoes and high heels (sometimes on surfaces like concrete) puts a much different stress on the spine than does natively walking barefoot on the earth.

In fact, no matter how much we might try to pay attention to health, it's difficult to foster a lifestyle that avoids spinal abnormalities. Regular chiropractic care is how we keep these abnormalities at bay.

From the Spine to the Body

Though physical subluxation is thought of as a mechanical, forceful event, there's even more to it than that. Chemical and biochemical stress often directly impact the nerves, making hardly-noticeable environmental interactions just as important as the more visible, physical lifestyle choices we make.

With so much of our daily lives affecting the spine, what exactly does that mean for health? As we've discussed, if you wait until symptoms to show up, it's often too late. A cascade of health issues may already be set in motion. Let's consider the sections of the spine, their neurology, and how abnormalities may affect the body.

Cervical

The pressure created by abnormalities at the top of the spine can affect the transition between the brainstem and spinal cord. The nervous system at this section is responsible for breathing, heart rate, and other subconscious functions of the body.

In 2007, researchers at the University of Chicago evaluated the effects of a single adjustment to the highest cervical vertebra. (ScienceDaily, 2007) Each of the 50 participants had both high blood pressure and an abnormality in the Atlas vertebra. This part of the neck can easily be out of alignment without any indication of pain.

The patients' blood pressure was checked right after the adjustment and again at eight weeks—and the results were phenomenal. Blood pressure reduction was similar to what might be expected from *two* different hypertension medications. From one adjustment! And eight weeks later, the results had continued.

In another study conducted in 2012, blood pressure was again monitored with a chiropractic adjustment of the cervical spine. This time, the hypotensive (low blood pressure) participants saw an increase in blood pressure. (Torns, 2012) Potentially, the effect of chiropractic on blood pressure could be normalizing, and the researchers called for a deeper look into this effect and its possible implications.

You see, chiropractic care isn't about forcing the body to express itself one way or another. There is no adjustment "for" high blood pressure any more than there is an adjustment "for" low blood pressure. **The adjustment is for the person, so that the body's own innate wisdom can better track towards what is normal for him or her.**

Other body functions connected to the cervical spine include: the muscles and circulation of the arms, elbows, and wrists; asthma and lung health; vision, headaches, and dizziness.

Thoracic

The next section of the spine is the largest and extends from the top of the shoulders to the mid-back. The nerves that run through the thoracic spine reach through the middle of the body. So the esophagus, lungs, and heart might be affected by both the cervical and thoracic spine, but in very different ways.

The thoracic spine connects nerves to the organs in the middle of the body— digestive system, adrenals, and uterus. For example, the nerves supplying the gallbladder and liver come through the hepatic plexus at T4-T9, as does the Vagus nerve through the upper cervical spine. (Keet, *The Pyloric Sphincteric Cylinder In Health and Disease*) Either of these nerve supplies can affect the gallbladder or liver, and an adjustment can be important when health is suffering in these ways.

In the '90s, researchers started to look into the idea that going to the chiropractor can keep you from getting sick. They measured physical responses, including white blood cell counts increasing after the adjustment, and had some ideas about how exactly the immune system might be responding to the subluxation and correction. (Brennan, et al, 1991)

From 2006-2010, Canadian researchers took a look again, with a single thoracic adjustment as the focus. They confirmed that in the right circumstances, the immune system can be directly and positively affected by chiropractic adjustments, reflected within cytokines, a specific component of the immune response. (Teodorczyk-Injeyan, et al, 2010) Their work continues, learning exactly how the process works and how we can utilize it most effectively. Our work is to do the adjustments and allow the benefits to take root. I can tell you that, personally, when I was a child, whenever I was run down, my chiropractor father would analyze my spine and, most often, adjust me. I would bounce back to health quicker than the other kids. Anecdotally, this is a trend nearly all chiropractors observe in their patients—and the research is starting to explain why.

Lumbar

Low in the back, the lumbar vertebrae are the last free-moving vertebrae in the spine, while the sacral and coccygeal sections are fused and extend into the buttocks. The buttocks, groin, thighs, and legs are anchored here, and the nerves that move through the lumbar spine affect lower intestines and reproductive organs.

Lower back pain is a common motivation for a chiropractic appointment, though even that is sometimes under-utilized. In pregnancy, for example, when that curve of your lower back is strained and causing pain, your care provider might not have much of an answer for you. Chiropractic, on the other hand, is a safe source of relief of that nagging, sometimes debilitating, lumbar-region pain, even in pregnancy. (Peterson, 2014)

A randomized, double-blind, controlled clinical trial evaluated the levels of pain in patients with problems in their lower back before and after a lumbar adjustment. Every indicator of pain improved for the treatment group, with no changes in the control group. (Vieira-Pellenz, 2014) If you're experiencing back pain at any level, but especially in the lower lumbar region, and you haven't yet visited a chiropractor, just about every piece of research I have seen would indicate that now is the time. Medication may be designed to block pain—but chiropractic is all about safely and effectively getting to the cause.

From a purely mechanical perspective, chiropractic care for lower back pain will typically include adjustments to these segments. But, don't forget those adjustments also have an impact on the organs you don't feel—not just the muscles and select nerves that you do feel.

Today's Research

Research is vital. Notably, I've learned in research seminars that approximately 18% of people are high fact-finders and cautious adopters. In a day when you have so many options in taking care of your health, I don't blame anyone for doing their homework and seeking out research to support their choices.

For the more-than 80% of the population that relies less heavily on statistics, the empirical evidence shines, and the principle makes sense. The outcomes are obvious. A mentor of mine, Dr. James W. Parker, who founded Parker University and its chiropractic programme, used to say "Chiropractic Works. It gets results. And that's what counts."

As the chiropractic profession forges forward in its own research to advance our understandings of what we've observed clinically for over 100 years, there are a few things everyone in that 18% should know.

First, there actually is a lot of research to support chiropractic. Dr. Deed Harrison is arguably the most published chiropractor ever, representing the Chiropractic Biophysics® Technique, the most published named chiropractic technique within the Index Medicus. Its non-profit organization's research centers around spinal biomechanics, ideal and average human alignment variables, posture modeling, and randomized and non-randomized trials evaluating technique outcomes.

The research coming out of the Centre for Chiropractic Research within the New Zealand College of Chiropractic is revealing some of the most comprehensive information about the role of the spine and its impact on the nervous system that we have seen to date. The Centre's Director of Research, Dr. Heidi Haavik, has conducted and published studies to demonstrate the connections between chiropractic care and asthma, blood pressure, and brain function. As a result, she has received numerous scholarships and countless awards. Dr. Haavik's ongoing research explores the impact of chiropractic care on the central nervous system, its ability to adapt to its environment, and human function and quality of life.

Nearly every chiropractic institution in North America possesses its own research department. Remarkably, some of what we are learning today comes out of non-chiropractic institutions (case in point, the blood pressure study referenced above). Pubmed returns over 7,000 studies pertaining to "chiropractic," with even more published on chiro.org. Entire journals are dedicated to this research, including the Annals of Vertebral Subluxation Research, the Journal of Manipulative and Physiological Therapeutics, and others.

Next, there is an assumed hierarchy of research, meaning that the double-blind, clinically-controlled, placebo-based trial has become the gold standard. This said, cohort studies, case studies, case reports, editorials, and even animal studies and in vitro studies are not invalid. They often contribute to the more rigorous, systematic reviews of all relevant data. Even more important, when we approach chiropractic from a philosophical standpoint, the concept of vitalism and Innate Intelligence *asks* different questions in research than does mechanism—and therefore leads to different types of outcomes and evidence. (Hawk, 2013)

The work of research has been done for years and continues in institutions to this day. So why aren't there more randomized trials and systematic reviews? There's no tactful way to say this, but drug companies fuel most of those studies while chiropractic institutions are working off funding from donors. The institutions often have different goals than the prominent funders, as well. When I was in school, I worked on a follow-up study to research that had identified an increase in CD4 (a type of white blood cell that fights infection) counts in HIV+ patients. (Hightower, 1994) As soon as this effect was realized, the study shifted to different types of outcome measures so that we could best refine the technique and get people the care they needed.

Finally, more research doesn't mean something will or won't work for you. Sometimes you have to do the research with yourself. And, through consideration of chiropractic's outstanding safety and track record and the fact that there are a growing number of methods in practice to support individual cases, even my friends who were classically opposed to referring to chiropractors are increasingly going themselves.

Chiropractic Could Be Your Missing Link

Changes to lifestyle, diet, stress, and sleep are important. Your efforts aren't lost in these areas, by any stretch. Take care of your body in any way that you can! But what happens when you've made the changes and still haven't seen the results you want? Many of you have been there—or may be there right now. Without results for your efforts, burnout is far more likely.

Chiropractic care could be the missing link. If you haven't yet evaluated your spine—and, by extension, your nervous system and muscular structure—it's time to make an appointment with a chiropractor.

At a chiropractic appointment, you might have specific adjustments based on an analysis of your health concerns or based on a physiological exam of your spine. (Likely, it will be a combination of both.) Your chiropractor might take x-rays for a closer look, or incorporate other forms of analysis; including video fluoroscopy, surface electromyography, spinal thermography, or computerized postural analysis.

The adjustment itself is usually a short appointment. Some tables are flat; others are in moving sections based on the needs of the adjustment and the preference of the doctor. Chiropractic adjustments are designed to correct areas of subluxation by using techniques of pressure ... to put it plainly: thrusting the spine very specifically at identified points. Sometimes this is done by hand and sometimes this is done with instruments and tools. Adjustment tables can be static or moving. Some adjustments are felt or even heard by the patient; others are not.

A qualified chiropractor has studied for years and must pass certification requirements, as well as maintain licensing. Chiropractors are primary care providers and are experts in their fields of study. The youngest babies and oldest family members are safe in the hands of a trained chiropractor and, as we have seen, stand to benefit much.

After the adjustment, your chiropractor will likely help you to make better lifestyle decisions. Personalized exercises and posture techniques—some using equipment and, others, just using your own body weight—can help to maintain the changes from the adjustment. Sometimes, as we saw with the hypertension study, one adjustment can do a great deal. Other times, a whole regimen and supporting lifestyle changes will be necessary. This kind of ongoing partnership with a chiropractor can form the cornerstone of a better life and a healthier family.

A New Understanding for the Whole Family

Kory Cobb

"

Three years ago, after having our fourth child, my baby and I were both doing terrible. Our little Annie would barely sleep—and that was only when she was on the corner of our sectional couch, wrapped in a soft blanket. After having three kids, you'd think I had it all figured out. But Annie was colicky, and I had no idea how to help her, or our family. The sleep deprivation for both of us wrecked me. The other kids really didn't have their mom—they had a postpartum mess, blubbering about, hollering commands, and trying to get everyone to play quietly so the baby could sleep.

A friend asked if we had considered "getting her adjusted." Not really knowing what that meant, I responded, "I would try anything at this point." Sensing that this was a good step to explore, I brought Annie to a local, family chiropractor whom I had met the year before. I had no idea what to expect, but within forty-eight hours of Annie receiving a gentle, pediatric chiropractic adjustment, alongside the introduction of some probiotics for her little gut— she was normal. From inconsolable screaming for over five hours per day to— normal. I was flabbergasted and relieved.

Talking things through with my new chiropractor, my eyes were opened to a whole new understanding of how God made our bodies. And, because Annie's birth had been difficult—she had been born "sunny side up"—it made sense that Annie's cervical spinal alignment had been compromised at birth.

The approach made sense. We decided to have our entire family evaluated, which made other things start to make sense too.

I had been experiencing tingling in my left arm and hand. After realizing that I had been holding and nursing a colicky baby most of the day and night, my thoracic and cervical spine were out of sorts and needed care.

My husband, who had been through five years of pain and was diagnosed with scapulothoracic bursitis, had been told that his only solution was to have surgery to "scrape" the muscle, with a good probability that the pain would return within a few years. After two months of chiropractic care, he was feeling normal and was in no pain whatsoever.

Our son, who had been on several antibiotics as a toddler, had a weak immune system and showed symptoms of Attention Deficit Disorder. But, after 6 weeks of chiropractic care, he was able to complete his homework in half the time. His behavior improved so much that he was awarded "Citizen of the Month!" His before and after X-ray results were dramatic; he had lost 73% of the natural curve in his neck, but this loss was reduced to only 18% by the time he had his first reassessment. Much else was measurably improved, as well!

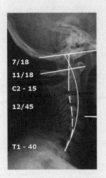

BEFORE

Prior to starting care, Eli's cervical lordosis (the natural curvature in the neck which should measure 45°) had been reduced to only 12°. The angles of measurement at the skull and at the first vertebra in the neck (which should both measure 18° with respect to the horizontal plane) measured only 7° and 11°.

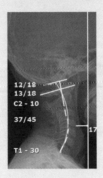

AFTER

Once starting care, Eli's cervical lordosis improved to 37°. The occiput and first cervical vertebra plane lines improved to 12° and 13°, respectively. Alongside these measurable changes, Eli's signs and symptoms improved dramatically, as well.

Lastly, our daughter Amelia had experienced intense emotional battles between the ages of four and six. For a couple years, we noticed that she would always sleep in the same position, face down with her head always to the one, same side. It made sense that this repeated torque in her neck would have affected the top of her spine, closest to the brain and brainstem. With exercises and specific adjustments to correct the imbalance in her neck, her emotional health has become more steady, making life for the family more enjoyable.

So often, we can be led to our wit's end before we make the decision to get better. I am so thankful my friend reaching out to me and that I was transparent enough to respond honestly. As a result, our family's life will never be the same. 🙶

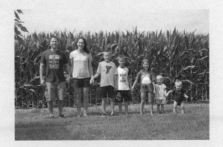

CHAPTER 4

Eat Well to Live Well

A balanced nervous system and healthy spine are at the core of MaxLiving's 5 Essentials. If you need a simple first step, that would be it. In essence, chiropractic care is about freeing your nervous system to *feed* your body the resources it needs to function as intended. But it cannot literally feed your body. The nervous system cannot "turn bacon into broccoli," as we say, so this brings us to the next essential: nutrition.

Throughout this chapter, we'll walk through the foundational nutrients our bodies need, the interference created by standard North American diets, and how we can reconcile our existing lifestyles to one of innate healing and the nutrition we need. Later, in the appendix, you'll find the Core and Advanced eating plans recommended throughout, as well as practical help like meal plans, recipes, and tips for navigating the grocery store. For now, let's spend some time building the foundation for those healthier habits.

A Brief History

Historically, people had little control over their diets. Aside from the most wealthy, whatever was regionally available was your diet by necessity. Agrarian societies grew what was favorable to their region. The more we centralized, food purchases could happen in the market, but the average person still had very little access to trade. Even as recently as the last couple of generations, the lack of refrigeration limited our ability to transport, mass-purchase, and store food.

In most ways, our modern access to all sorts of food has been an incredible development in human history. We know more now about the micronutrients our bodies need, as well as the foods in which they are abundant. Most households have access to those foods. But this new, broad access and our growing, nuanced understandings have led to a new problem: **No one can agree on what we should eat.**

We're now inundated with pyramids, plates, plans, and portions. The most recent shifts in diet philosophy are on the right track. More and more, people are adopting the philosophy that our bodies are meant to work properly in the first place, and we just need to get out of the way.

Primal, paleo, ancestral, blood type diets—they all insinuate that the body's natural design should be honored in whatever diet we follow. But with so many voices shouting about what's best, it's difficult to know which one is right. *Is* there one that's right? The confusion all too easily gives way to frustration, and when it does, massive processed, fast-food industries are there to break the fall.

Sugar

It's easy enough for diet plans and food gurus to tell you to avoid sugar. We can talk all day long about the evils of sugar—and we will get into some of those specifics in a moment, to be sure. But let's be very clear about it: sugar itself is not a source of interference. Our bodies are wired to handle a reasonable amount of bioavailable sugar. We need those good fruits and starches that have been part of the human diet from the very beginning.

The *interference* of sugar has taken many forms over those years, however, and has wreaked havoc on health. Completely divorced from naturally-occurring sugars, "sugar" as the ingredient we know cannot be found in nature. Even the least refined sugars are still refined in some way, so that there is now a spectrum of sugars to choose from—or, better yet, to avoid. (See Appendix C for some label-reading guidance and grocery store simplification.)

In its lower stages of refinement, sugar might come from the sugarcane plant and be processed into light brown crystals. Or, that same sugar can be stripped of the minerals (molasses is the byproduct of this process) and then bleached to be completely white—and completely devoid of nutrients. All along this spectrum, we find turbinado sugar, brown sugar, low-refinement sugar, and so on until there's simply white, refined sugar found in our pantries and in countless products on the market today. This sugar is a source of interference.

Jump past that level of refinement and into high fructose corn syrup, and the interference skyrockets. Sugar cane doesn't grow well in North America, but corn is prolific. **We consume more sugar from corn than from any other source, thanks in part to its many forms.** You're probably aware that you can't simply press, cook, or extract from an ear of corn until sugar or syrup emerges. Actual, molecular-level changes have to happen. The corn is milled into starch, then broken down with an enzyme at multiple stages, more and more until the glucose is converted to fructose in designer balances for varying degrees of sweetness. It's unrecognizable as a food, both to our eyes and our digestive tracts.

Growing Interference

Over the last three or four decades, the US government increasingly favored domestic corn over sugar imports. If you were an adult or even a child in the 1970s and '80s, you'll have noticed the shift in food over the years. From the volumes of sugar to the variances, our grocery stores, ads, and meals don't look the same anymore. In 1980, Coca-cola boasted 9 teaspoons of sugar in a can.

By 2006, Baskin-Robbins heir John Robbins turned down his rights to the company and instead wrote a book, *Healthy at 100*, warning us that "The average American consumes 53 teaspoons of sugar per day." (Robbins, 2006) Today, with sugar from all sources included, that number might even be low. In 2014, the New York City municipal government proclaimed that the average daily consumption is 93 packets, thanks to the standard North American diet and due to sugar being in— well, *everything.* (CB13Q, 2013)

Corn is so available and variations of corn syrup so cheap, it's increasingly difficult to avoid. Meanwhile, researchers recently uncovered a trail of sugar-lobby funding for studies beginning in the 1960s and onward. (Kearns, 2016) These studies were targeted at the vilification of fats. If you've wondered why diet recommendations have fluctuated so wildly from year to year, this is a good start. As fat became singled out for heart disease, the landscape of food options shifted heavily toward processed carbs and sugars.

Today, a similar pattern has emerged. As people become more unsettled with sugar and high-fructose corn syrup, corporations have scrambled to hold onto their product market. Artificial sweeteners are on the rise, further entrenching North American diets in highly-processed, highly unstable foods. We'll look closer at that shift when we talk about toxins and chemicals.

Low-fat—and now, low-sugar—food products are often heavily processed. The low-fat products often contain added sugar and the low-sugar products often contain carcinogenic chemicals.

Refined grains aren't technically sugar, but they might as well be. The processing process for flours and grains strips the minerals and nutrients that our bodies would otherwise need to use those foods efficiently. This includes the obvious culprits like white flour, white sugar, and junk food, and extends much further than many of us realize—corn flakes, white rice, even those chunky, "multi-grain" breads can be problematic.

Almost as soon as refined grains hit your mouth, they are broken down into simple sugars and, to our digestive systems, are little more than additions to our growing daily sugar count.

As the adage goes: **The whiter the bread, the quicker you're dead.**

The Consequences of Weight Gain

North America has busily chased low-fat diets, the high-sugar, high-carb alternatives—with increasingly sedentary lives—and it's done us no favors. Since the 1970s, childhood obesity has tripled. (CDC, 2017) According to the CDC, more than a third of adults in the US classify as obese. (CDC, 2017) Along with these increases has come the correlated concerns of heart disease, diabetes, and cancer. Less obvious but still significant connections have been made between sugar intake and inflammatory disease, cognitive dysfunction, and immune weakness.

An entire group of risk factors has been placed under the umbrella term *metabolic syndrome*. (AHA, 2015) If any three of the five risk factors are present (high glucose, low "good" cholesterol, high "bad" cholesterol, excessive waist circumference, or high blood pressure), metabolic syndrome is diagnosed and the chances of diabetes, stroke, and more go through the roof. More than thirty million Americans meet these qualifications, keeping heart disease as the top cause of death in the US year after year. (CDC, 2017)

Again—naturally-occurring sugars are part of traditional and healthy diets and can be used efficiently by the body. The interference of sugar refinement and excessive amounts of simple sugars in the diet create a very different digestive process. Where the body is adept at using the foods we eat to produce energy and circulate nutrients, it's only prepared to circulate a minimal amount of sugar in the bloodstream at any given time to convert it to energy.

When we surpass that level, insulin production from the pancreas signals cells in the liver and muscles to allow glucose in for storage. Some amount of energy storage is good, but when we overload the system entirely, storage is shifted to fat stores. If it continues, there's a greater risk of insulin resistance—the body no longer listening to the signals and being unable to convert or remove sugar from the bloodstream—and eventual type 2 diabetes. (NIH, 2009)

The Worst News

No one wants to be diagnosed with disease, but when we're entrenched in this lifestyle, it becomes all too commonplace. How often do we discuss the perils of aging in our society? Creaky knees, a growing stack of prescriptions, and a laundry list of diagnoses? The number of diabetic and pre-diabetic people in the developed world continues to grow, and as long as we continue to wear our bodies down, it won't stop.

But the most dreaded diagnosis comes in the form of cancer.

Today, we'd be hard-pressed to find someone who hasn't been affected by cancer directly or within their circle of friends and family members. We know for sure that certain cancers are more likely to show up in certain diets (look for the discussion on processed meats in a few pages). So the question remains: can we prevent or eliminate cancer with diet? And, specifically, by controlling sugar intake?

In 1931, the Warburg hypothesis won Otto Warburg the Nobel Prize in Physiology or Medicine. Building on the idea that the body's cells grow in the presence of food—specifically, triggered by Insulin-like Growth Factor (IGF-1) when blood sugar increases—Professor Warburg hypothesized that cancer cells would do the same. Since they have eight times the receptors for IGF-1 than healthy body cells, it stands to reason that tumors would respond in kind, and much faster. Researchers like Lewis Cantley have led the resurgence in understanding the Warburg effect and the connection between metabolism and cancer, maintaining that, *"Understanding this important aspect of biology is likely to have a major impact on our understanding of cell proliferation control and cancer."* (Heiden, Cantley, Thompson, 2009)

Other researchers, while acknowledging the advancements that Professor Warburg's observations have led us toward, note that it's still a hypothesis and might not be our be-all, end-all answer for cancer causation. (Liberti, Locasale, 2013) More questions have been raised than answered, and the research journey continues on.

While we don't have data solid enough to tell us whether a certain diet will cure cancer or eliminate our risks, we can all agree that the body constantly tries to eliminate mutated, cancerous cells, and certain lifestyles can make those existing processes more labored and ineffective. **Although our normal body processes remove cancerous cells constantly, day and night, we have to allow them to do so.** The same immune system that clears the body of infectious disease removes cancer cells by the thousands. When we eat a poor diet—specifically, sugar and refined grains that turn into sugar and put a strain on our metabolic resources—we're bogging down the system.

Research is advancing every day, and our understanding of this blight will be even greater in the next generation than when Professor Warburg won the Nobel. Regardless of the eventual outcome, do we really want to build on our health risks for the sake of a simple sugar habit? Much like our spinal health, if we wait for the consequences to appear, it will be too late.

Knowing that your body needs better foods to thrive and—quite literally—survive, it's important start to make changes now, before the effects begin to add up.

Fat

Our society clearly nurtures a love/hate relationship with fat. There are now at least 15,000 different "low-fat" products on the shelves of our grocery stores, and with no improvement in health to show for it. Fat content dropped, simple-sugar content jumped, and obesity ran rampant. We're still battling obesity today more than ever, and with it, heart disease.

When I was writing about this topic years ago, the American Heart Association had consistently recommended a 2,000 calorie, low-fat diet. Today, the standard has only shifted slightly, to include low-fat dairy, nuts, and specifically non-tropical vegetable oils—so peanut and canola oils are recommended over coconut oil based purely on their content of saturated fat. (AHA, 2017)

Could it be that the problem is not with adherence to these plans but with the plans themselves?

In spite of decades of low-fat messages and calorie-counting paradigms, mortality rates from heart disease, diabetes, and cancer have continued to climb. (Ford, Capewell, 2007) All too often, we're told that losing weight is "simple math": lower calorie intake and higher calorie output. Eat less and move more. But our bodies are anything but simple.

By assuming all fats are made equal and can equally damage the body, we've starved ourselves of a vital nutrient. **Some fats are absolutely necessary, and without them, the body has to accommodate for the loss.**

This is another area where primal or innate diets have gotten it right. Consider the Inuit diets that relied so heavily on the fats from fish and seals, or the conceptualized diet of nuts and seeds and animal protein of a hunter/gatherer. The more traditional a diet becomes, the more we see healthy fats are included. Cavemen might have had a lot of threats, but obesity and heart disease weren't likely on the list.

Cholesterol

Public health campaigns often center around the theory that cholesterol comes from fat and then leads to heart disease. Known as the lipid hypothesis, it's still largely questionable, especially with long-term research.

The lipid hypothesis has permeated medical philosophies as long ago as Chinese texts. As always, a hypothesis should be open to further review, and this one just doesn't hold up. In 2015, the USDA dropped it's low-cholesterol diet recommendations because *high cholesterol foods do not elevate your cholesterol.* (USDA, 2015) There is simply no available evidence to justify this concern.

Even if we were to play devil's advocate and say that high cholesterol foods could have an impact on serum cholesterol, having high cholesterol itself is not the cause of heart disease. As a person gets older, cholesterol actually appears to drop off entirely as a correlated factor for all-cause or cardiovascular mortality. (Ravnskov, et al, 2016) Another study, evaluating a specific population's health risks and total cholesterol, acknowledged that findings seem to be inconsistent across the board. Some correlate low cholesterol with mortality while others say high cholesterol is the risk. (Bae, 2012)

The cholesterol connection is simply inconsistent on its own. Instead, we need to look at the whole picture—our food source and consumption, lifestyle and habits, movement and metabolism—to determine risk and return.

How the Body Uses Fats

Fat doesn't make you fat. Your inability to burn fat is what makes you fat. The burning of body fat is a function of hormones, primarily *leptin*, which is regulated by the fat cells themselves. Functioning properly, leptin tells your brain when you're full, when to use fat for energy, and when to eat more. This would have been an incredibly helpful gauge in those cavemen days, when your body stored energy for days and weeks in the absence of food and would need an urgency trigger when the stores were running low.

In the absence of survival in the wild, leptin is more or less a bored troublemaker, causing problems. Its intended, beneficial effects are misplaced in the average North American lifestyle, leading to weight gain and broken relationships with food. Even worse, our periods of absence and starvation are not a measure of food availability but *nutrient* availability. Calorie limitation can deprive the body of nutrients and, as a 2015 study summarized, is a "self-imposed, voluntary famine." (Macpherson-Sánchez, 2015)

Even when we aren't limiting intake, however, a lack of nutrients can signal famine just as much as a lack of food. **The body doesn't recognize intake as much as it recognizes nutrients.**

While our bodies perceive starvation in the absence of intake, nutrients, or both, leptin stashes fat away. Often, the pseudo-starvation effect also signals to the brain that we feel full and can keep on surviving anyway. Meanwhile, we keep feeding it unrecognizable, empty foods, and the cycle goes on until leptin receptors are completely burned out and the body stops communicating about fat regulation altogether. Despite high leptin levels, your body's ability to burn fat becomes impaired. (Are you sensing a pattern, here? This is a cycle not unlike insulin resistance and diabetes.)

We're starving for nutrients, good fats among them. But when I say *good* fats, I really mean *great.* The function of essential fatty acids is vital for brain function, and it's not something for which the body can compensate if we aren't consuming them in the diet. And when I say *bad* fats, I really mean *damaged* fats. Because the fats we consider to be bad are usually unnaturally extracted, modified, or processed into something else entirely. Remember this: **Damaged fats damage the body.**

Healthy fats form the vast majority of brain tissue and are vital for cognitive function in adults and brain development in children. They also lower inflammation and build cell membranes, reducing pain and aiding in the communication between cells and nerves. In other words, fats optimize your body's electrical mechanisms. Not to mention the fat layers themselves. We need some amount of fat in our bodies to cushion organs and insulate against temperature changes. And, as something of an organ itself, fatty tissue regulates hormones.

Interestingly, the brain—composed of nearly 60% fat content and craving most of the healthy fats you'll consume—can't actually absorb fat directly. (Chang, Ke, Chen, 2009) (Fan, 2013) The liver works to convert fat intake and fat storage into ketones, which feed the brain the energy it needs. So not only do you have to ingest the right nutrients, but your body has to be functioning properly in order to convert those nutrients into usable forms. An extremely high-fat, low-carb diet ("keto" diets) is intended to jumpstart that process to feed the brain and anti-inflammatory signals directly, since ketones become primary fuel during starvation.

Though the low-fat, low-calorie chronic dieter will be drawn to the perceived freedom of going full-tilt with bacon, it's not always as easy as it sounds. Starvation is starvation, and there are drawbacks to depriving your body of the carbohydrates it's used to consuming. You might "run" into bathroom issues. The brain-fuel might turn into brain-fog as vitamin stores drop. You could—strange as it may seem—grow tired of all those bun-less buffalo burgers and avocados. It's little wonder that a supplement market for instant, effortless ketosis has opened up. Who doesn't love the idea that you could keep your current lifestyle, add a supplement, then suddenly lose fat stores while feeding your brain?

But we aren't here to rely on something made in a factory. We aren't looking for another silver bullet to do the work for us. We only need to get out of the way of our normal body processes. We must remove the interference of damaged fats, starvation-modes, and fat storage.

Building a Better Relationship with Fats

Eating fat to lose fat is appealing and not without its merits, but we aren't concerned about surface results alone. We are digging deep to restore the essentials, and in this case, that means creating a better relationship with dietary fats.

Not all fats are created equal—and that's a rather literal statement! The molecular structure of fats varies, which is where we get the terms *saturated, unsaturated,* and *trans-fats.* They refer to the way the carbon chains connect and become saturated with hydrogen, identifiable by their behavior at room temperature. You've no doubt heard and used these terms, but let's reiterate and put them under the lens of MaxLiving principles. Case in point: the coconut oil *controversy.*

If you hadn't read the 2017 warning published by the American Heart Association, you're probably confused by that statement. (Sacks, 2017) *Who could possibly be confused by coconut oil?* But it's true—coconut oil was lumped in with any old saturated fat and considered problematic. The headlines went wild. It's a symptom of our studies and recommendations painting with broad strokes and lumping the good in with the bad.

In a world where all saturated fats are unhealthy and all unsaturated fats are preferred, coconut oil is a heart risk while distorted, highly-processed canola oil is a better option. I don't know about you, but I wouldn't function well in that world!

Now, you can undoubtedly find people to say whatever you want to hear about fats. Just as we see with philosophies of health in general, if the underlying paradigm is flawed, the application will be faulty. Add to that a clickbait-heavy "journalistic" society that runs faulty conclusions to their extremes, and it's little wonder consumers are confused.

This is why I recognize that there is not one diet that suits all people. This is also why I consider the MaxLiving approach to diet and nutrition to be a framework and not prescriptive. And yes, I could give you a gamut of tests to run to identify your most ideal nutritional requirements, but I'll also tell you to make logical steps toward health then listen to your body. I do believe, in your core, your body knows what is best—and you can be in tune with its wishes.

In other words, it's not about creating more villains and heroes, silver bullets and one-size-fits-all fixes. The MaxLiving view of health is about feeding our bodies the things it needs and not impeding one's innate functions.

Eliminating Fat Interference

Fat interference can come in many forms:

- A high-fat, high-toxin, low-movement lifestyle
- Healthy fats that are otherwise damaged
- Fats that are processed into non-foods (hydrogenated oils, trans fats)

We've already talked about how even good fats cannot fix a bad diet—we cannot just add coconut oil and expect everything to be better. But there's also the matter of healthy fats, within a healthy lifestyle, that become damaged before consumption.

Rancid Oils

Labeling laws do not require much in the way of rancidification. At any point during manufacture, storage, and home-use, oils can become oxidized and rancid. The most "healthy" of oils are most subject to this kind of damage. Saturated fats—butter and coconut oil included, identifiable by becoming solid at room temperatures—are by default more stable as they structurally adapt to changing environments. Unsaturated fats—olive oil and grapeseed oil, for example— remain liquid and are sensitive to air, heat, and light. This is why your olive oil should come in a dark bottle and not be used for pan-frying.

Sourcing, storage, and use of healthy, unsaturated oils becomes important. The company or farm should be reputable, paying close attention to bottling times and methods. Mass-production of specialized oils is hardly reliable—by the time it makes it from farm to processing to shipping to your door, has it been in transit long enough to go rancid? Probably, and it isn't worth the risk to your health.

Damaged oils are interference in all forms. The oxidation splits otherwise stable chains of fat molecules into free radicals, which continue the oxidation process. Free radicals, you might be aware, are directly connected to cancer. Even if this problem were eliminated, the damage to the food structure renders the fat as something unrecognizable to the body. As much as we need to be concerned about sugar as it relates to both cancer and inflammatory disease, today's research is showing just as many signs that damaged fats are an enemy that can't be overlooked. (Grootveld, et al, 2001)

Trans Fats

We're already aware of the non-nutrient "foods" that comes in the form of processed, packaged products, and the damaged fats found in them are a significant reason why. Ironically, these "foods" are valued for their shelf-stability—they won't go rancid easily, at least!—but the trans fats and hydrogenated oils found in these foods are damaged from the get go.

The worst culprits are partially hydrogenated (trans fats) and hydrogenated oils, formed when hydrogen molecules are forced into unsaturated fats to create more saturation and shelf-stabilization. In other words, they are completely restructured into something the body doesn't recognize. For the most part, society agrees that trans fats are bad, with many products and restaurants bragging about being trans-fat-free.

Unfortunately, not only are they still prevalent in candies and packaged junk food, but labeling requirements haven't caught up. A product can be "trans-fat-free" if the trans fat content is less than 500 mg per serving. (FDA, 2017) Factor in deceptive serving sizes on the labels, and consumers are unquestioningly consuming more trans fats than they realize, even when trying to avoid them. With trans fats posing a greater risk of heart disease than saturated fats, it's little wonder heart disease is so prevalent. (Science Daily, 2015)

Processed Vegetable Oil

Extracted from their plants of origin, vegetable oils are heavy in omega-6 fatty acids. Even without hydrogenation, vegetable oils are abundant in our grocery stores, restaurants, and recipes, providing the Standard American Diet with nearly unlimited sources of omega-6 fats. Ideally, omega-6 intake should fall somewhere between a 1:1 and a a 4:1 ratio compared with omega-3 consumption. Thanks to extracted oils and imbalanced diets, North Americans might consume as much as 50:1 omega 6 to omega 3 fats. Far too many of us have these imbalances to thank for inflammation, obstructed circulation, and more.

There are plenty of healthy, delicious vegetable oils to enjoy in your diet, but be aware of how they traveled from farm to table. Cold-pressed oils are closest to nature, retaining their original molecular structures. In this form, there are few oils you need to avoid. But there is a spectrum of processing to be aware of—from cold pressed, to pressed, to the eventual step of deodorization, which turns the flavor bland and allows for higher heat cooking. At that stage, every oil has a bit of trans fat, whether or not it's labeled, and it's the most common form of non-descript "vegetable oil" or canola oil.

In its natural state, cold-pressed canola oil is not a bad option. But that's not what stocks our unhealthy pantries and fries up chicken in commercial, deep-fat (troublingly oxidized) fryers. (Crosby, 2017) In Appendix C, we've put together a list of fats to look for and damaged fats to avoid.

The fats that the body cannot use—damaged, unrecognizable, and stacked into an unhealthy lifestyle—are left through the body like damage in the wake of a storm. Cell membranes, fat stores, and arterial walls are all at risk, and that baked treat or greasy snack will not be worth the cost.

Non-Foods

The running theme here is simple: our bodies expect food in a certain state, and when we tamper with that process, we tamper with our health. The alterations might be progressive—as with sugar's gradual descent into HFCS—or sudden. They might transform the food entirely—as with hydrogenated oils—or they might be invisible. No matter the interference, from toxins to trans fats to refinement and additions, our bodies have to deal with these components as something other than food.

Even though we think of food as whatever we eat, our bodies can only deal in nutrients and waste. Everything comes from somewhere and everything must be broken down into something else. No individual food—whether whole and healthy or an un-food—goes without its effects on the body.

It's unfortunate that we have to label any food "organic". By nature, food *should* be an organic item, as opposed to inorganic, non-living matter. But given the kinds of toxins we're dealing with, the moniker is appropriate. When Rachel Carson wrote *Silent Spring* in the 1960s, the US was dumping more than six-hundred-*million* pounds of pesticides indiscriminately throughout neighborhoods, roadsides, and in aerial sprays. (Encyclopedia.com, 2017) Hundreds of the chemicals poured into and around communities were completely untested. Her writings brought attention to the gross negligence of these campaigns—asking her readers to imagine the stark reality of a spring without chirping birds or the buzz of bees—and went a long way toward curbing such rampant use of toxins.

But the spraying hasn't stopped. It's only moved into low-visibility areas, leaving our major crops doused in chemical poison and the soil stripped of its nutrients. And approved chemicals are still largely untested. Approximately 3,000 additives, preservatives, and colorings are FDA approved—but do we know how they alter the nutrient content of the food we eat? (FDA, 2017) **Not all toxins lead to death, but they all inhibit a healthy life.**

Food might stray from its original form if the soil has little nutrients to imbue. It will be weakened and carry toxic residue if it's sprayed at the soil with herbicides, on the vine with pesticides, or with fungicides as a preservative. It will lose nutrient content and carry un-food additives if it's altered and processed in a factory. It will grow old and further degrade as it travels hundreds of miles to wait on a grocery store shelf. **The further food moves from its original form, the less your body will recognize it as a food.**

Some of it will be detoxed out through our livers. Some of it will stay largely undigested in unusable "food" and pass right through the body. But some of it, having nowhere else to go, will be stored in the safest place our body can think of: fat tissue.

A diet filled with low-fat, low-sugar non-food is also laced with additives for flavor to make up for all the fat it's missing, and artificial sweeteners that keep us coming back for more. All of those chemicals, not to mention the pesticides, packaging, and general environmental toxins we face every day, are stored and stashed in our bodies. Ironically, well-intended efforts to eliminate fat could be keeping us from losing weight (and keeping it off), feeling good, thinking well, or all of the above.

Toxins are fat soluble more than water soluble, which means what can't be sweat out or excreted in some way will be tucked into the pads of fat we hoped to lose with all those low-fat, no-sugar products. But while adipose tissue serves to stash away toxins to keep them from circulating in the bloodstream, lipophilic toxins can technically make it to any fatty tissue in the body. And where else might that be? There's fat lining your nerves, fat making up your brain, and fat being broken down through the liver and digestive tract.

In the search for better prevention and resolution for the obesity epidemic, researchers have tuned into this connection to see what we can discover about toxicity and weight gain. Certain endocrine-disrupting chemicals have been categorized as *obesogenic* due to their recurring correlation with weight gain. The evidence is still mounting, and the resulting theory is called the obesogenic hypothesis, indicating toxic exposure ranging from organochlorines to BPA and phthalates as instigators of weight gain or potentially restricting weight loss. For example, one review of the most recent obesogenic findings notes that circulating levels of BPA were connected with increased levels of leptin and ghrelin, both of which serve to modulate hunger cues. (Darbre, 2017)

As the evidence continues to mount for the specific actions of these persistent chemicals in our bodies, one thing is clear: the continued accumulation of fat-soluble toxins will always be a problem within the body. It's our job to eliminate that interference with our choices, habits, and lifestyle.

Dangerous from Growth Stages

The first and most obvious concern we have with toxic foods begins with pesticide use in the growth stages. **By design, pesticides are meant to be toxic**. Not only are they effective in their job to eliminate insects, weeds, and any pest presence in food production, but they are known to be dangerous to humans. Dose-dependency only applies to how quickly and shockingly the poison affects you. No one would drink it. Hardly anyone would spray or apply it without protective gear. So why do we eat pounds of food laden with pesticide residue every single day?

The Pesticide Action Network of North America (PANNA) has detected dozens of different exposures per person, every day, through food alone and notes that the American Academy of Pediatricians (AAP) cites food as a child's most frequent exposure to pesticides. (PANNA, 2017) And this is all without mentioning the cleaning products, body care products, and other sources of toxins in the home and school and workplace.

Pesticides don't come on labels, so we rely on "organic" qualifications to direct us away from as many of these toxins as possible. Growth-enhancers are used in livestock to keep up with the sheer volume of demand. Chickens, cattle, and pork are grown with steroids and fed fattening, toxin-sprayed grains to help them reach peak development fast enough for North American demand to be satisfied. Tight growth spaces and unhealthy animals require constant disease control, so regular antibiotics are a staple, as well.

Once you remember that toxins are stored in fat—marbled and laced throughout most meat products—you can see why organically-pastured animals are vital for healthy meat sources.

Problematic Processing

Eliminating or minimizing toxins in the foods that still look like food—choosing organic produce, sourcing meat well—can be challenging enough. Once food becomes processed into a new, packaged food, your chances of avoiding toxins or un-food are slim to none. Some of that is the nature of preservation. If you expect something to be completely shelf-stable and ready in your grocer's snack aisle, you'll be stuck with preservatives and stabilizing additives. Some of the additions, however, are insidious and difficult to spot.

Nitrites are another good example of hidden, less-than-obvious additives. Most commonly, nitrites are added to packaged meat—deli slices and sausages, and also soups and frozen foods containing meat. In 2009, the World Cancer Research Fund advised a limit of red meat at less than 11 oz. (cooked weight) per week, with "very little, if any of which to be processed." Over seven years, an extensive study tracked 200,000 people to find that the people who consumed meats with nitrites regularly saw a 68% increase in risks of pancreatic cancer. (Nöthlings, et al, 2005) It's not necessarily meat alone that's a problem, either, but the carcinogenic substances related to preparation. Their findings also included some interesting caveats that we can learn from in our everyday meal-planning and food choices:

1. Both red and processed meat intakes were associated with an increased risk of pancreatic cancer.
2. Fat and saturated fat were deemed not likely to contribute to the underlying carcinogenic factors.
3. Carcinogenic substances related to meat preparation methods might be responsible for the 68% association.

Other health risks associated with meat production and consumption include cancers of the bowels, esophagus, stomach, endometrium, bladder, breast, and prostate, as well as type 2 diabetes, obesity, hypertension, and arthritis. (OMNICS, 2017)

Solutions

We know that today's sugar inhibits our body's natural processes. We know that damaged fats are inherently harmful. We know that toxins, processed junk, and non-foods are wasting valuable processes in our bodies. But what do we *do* with that information in our lives and for our families? **The MaxLiving Core Nutrition Plan builds on the awareness we have of dietary interference to create a practical plan that anyone can follow.** In my opinion, it is something everyone should.

For more targeted weight loss, internal restoration, and specific health and fitness goals, consider the Advanced plan. The Core Plan is designed to be flexible in everyday life. The Advanced Plan becomes less flexible, in that a few of your food options are removed from the list. But when you eat well, following a framework like the Core Plan, and still find yourself sluggish, ill, or inflamed, a period of stricter, more specific eating habits may be necessary.

Without verging into a clinical use of food as medicine, we have to understand that by the time we see symptoms, the damage has long been done. Sometimes, "just" removing interference actually looks like a lot of targeted work.

In this case, we're looking at conditions that have accumulated from years of various interferences. Toxins have stacked up, inflammation is out of control, hormones are out of whack, the body has forgotten how to use fat, and the brain is starved for energy. This might look like cognitive dysfunctions such as ADHD, metabolic syndrome illnesses like obesity and diabetes. It might mean fibromyalgia, autoimmune disorders, food intolerance, even cancer.

At the end of the book, you'll find both of the plans as well as specific recipes, meal plans, and shortcuts to be able to take these concepts from theory to application. If you're switching from the standard North American diet to the Core Plan, you'll undoubtedly feel better. But as you can see, it's a loosely-based eating plan— based on the highest-quality offerings—that you can adjust to your preferences and life. It's not a rigid diet.

As you build out your nutrition plans, consider the sources of your ingredients as carefully as you can. What kind of oil are the nuts cooked in? How have things been grown or processed? How close are you to the source, and do you know how to store it properly? Take what you know of each level and type of interference, and make better and better decisions for your family over time. You have to start somewhere, and this food plan will get you there.

Let's look quickly at some of the plan categories and important things to know, before digging into practical application.

High Level Nutrition

We've taken our nutritional knowledge and years of work with patients to create a Core Plan that's practical for just about everybody.

The Advanced Plan follows a similar structure, with some modifications for more specific goals. On this focus level, you'll need to *increase* your intake of healthy fats, *moderate* your intake of protein, and *eliminate* sugars, grains, and higher-sugar fruits. The goal will be to retrain your body to use fat as fuel, limit inflammation, and restore cell membrane function. As we walk through each category, I'll note significant differences between the plans. But for specific food lists, see the appendices, meal plans, and food lists in the back of the book.

Macronutrients as the Framework

Fats and proteins are the centerpieces of both plans, with excellent sources as the focus. Avoid damaged fats in all forms, and make sure your protein sources are as high-quality as possible. Make sure nuts and seeds are not cooked in damaged or processed oils. The Advanced Plan option will eliminate grains and pseudograins (such as quinoa) for potentially increased inflammation, and not only sugar but those higher-sugar fruits and anything else that converts quickly to sugar—more on this below. The Advanced Plan will also will moderate intake of protein. Feeding the body too much protein can cause problems with insulin, just like sugar. In place of the decreased protein, increase healthy fats.

Carbohydrates are just as vital, as long as they are chosen carefully. On all plans, avoid refined grains and most simple sugars, choosing fruits and vegetables that are high in fiber and low on the glycemic index. On the Advanced Plan, you'll increase high-fiber consumption throughout the whole day. These should comprise most of your carb and energy intake. The fruits that will become your best friends (generally, before lunch only) are berries, granny smith apples, lemons, limes, and grapefruits. Always consume with fat and fiber to buffer the impact of any sugars you may consume.

Meat

With vegans on one side and paleo on the other, we're constantly pulled between extremes. What we've found is: as long as you are obtaining the nutrients you need—including plenty of good fats—on the Core Plan, meat consumption is largely optional. Just because certain animal proteins are listed in the food guide presented, it does not mean that you *have* to eat them to be following the Core Plan. **The MaxLiving approach to eating isn't exclusively vegan, vegetarian, or carnivorous.**

The real challenge that comes with meat consumption is that its problems are invisible. It's one thing to avoid processed food products. It's quite another to analyze a display of meats that all look the same. Organically, sustainably grown meats might be more expensive, too. It's a commitment and a hassle. But if you're going to eat meat, the hassle is worth it.

Fish are among the healthiest types of meat, in theory, but once they have been farmed, all of that changes. Fish farms are often laden with disease and parasites. They are typically fed conventional grains, unnatural to their required diets. And the whole farm might be doused in chemicals in order to keep health problems at bay. (Seafood Watch, 2017) Instead, look for wild-caught or—when absolutely necessary—sustainably-grown fish. Better yet, avoid heavily-farmed species like tilapia and catfish altogether. They tend to have higher omega-6 ratios, with Atlantic salmon and trout faring much better. (Roizen, 2008)

Red meat gets a bad rap as being bad for you, but as always, there's more to the story. For one thing, people who choose not to eat red meat—vegetarians and pescatarians, especially—are usually more health conscious. (Akther, 2016) That difference in lifestyle can skew comparisons and the resulting data.

Another important qualifier is the difference between grass-fed, organically raised beef and conventionally-farmed options. Cattle are meant to forage greens, and interfering in that process alters the nutritional profile of the finished product. Grass-fed beef has better omega-6 to omega-3 ratios, and higher vitamin content, including twice the riboflavin, and three times the thiamine than grain-finished.

(Elswyk, McNeill, 2014) When beef is grain-finished—a commercial farming trick that keeps production moving quickly—never mind grain-fed for their entire lives, the cows are outside of their nutritional norm. Their bodies can't handle it, and often, they'd die early of acidosis if not for the slaughter. Mass-production cattle farms are harsh on the environment, hard on the cows, and provide a lesser food.

Vegetarian eating, while manageable nutritionally, does usually limit access to B12 vitamins. If it's a question of nutrition alone and not dietary preference or philosophical beliefs, the protein, mineral, and vitamin content in sustainably grown, grass-fed beef can bolster an already healthy diet.

On the other hand, if you're only eating a diet full of meats and low in vegetables, you're missing out on fiber and antioxidants. Listen to your body and be open to shifting your diet to get more of what you need when you need it.

Pork and Shellfish

First and foremost, many religions exclude the consumption of pork, shellfish, and other specific foods, and if that's your belief system, please honor it! Interestingly enough, the more we learn about the "unclean" versus "clean" animals, the more it makes logical sense to avoid them. Beef and lamb, clean animals in most faith traditions, are rudimentary animals, with extensive digestive systems and a basic diet of grass, grass, and more grass. Pork, shellfish, and catfish—usually designated as unclean—are bottom feeders or extremely tolerant of "slop" diets. They are biological compost bins.

Science tends to stand behind the cautions, especially once pork becomes processed into other food products. When the World Health Organization gathered experts to discuss the carcinogenic potential in processed meat, they found that a single hot dog or four strips of bacon every day could increase the risk of colorectal cancer by 18%. (WHO, 2015)

These foods are far from traditional in most cultures, and we are still learning where the exact risks might lie for unprocessed pork, shellfish, and other "unclean" foods. If you're still open to them until more conclusive evidence is found, that's certainly your choice. As with all foods and especially meat, know your source and your farm well. The cleaner they are raised, the better off you will be.

Soy

Soy tops the charts for hyperbole. You might hear it touted as a miracle food or lambasted as a masculinity-killer or a carcinogen. And it's not just what's taken out of context. The journals are full of studies that seem to contradict each other. (He, Chen, 2013) Before you decide whether or how to consume soy, you should understand what it is.

Fresh soybeans still in the pod (edamame) can be boiled or steamed and eaten as-is. Soy can also be fermented and formed into pastes, cakes, and sauces. Tempeh, miso, natto, and soy sauce fall in this category, while tofu is curdled rather than fermented. Identifying the kind of soy a study or expert is referring to can help decipher the application. Fermentation, as a rule, changes the composition of a food in natural ways, often doing the work that our bodies would have had to do while creating a more digestible and usable food.

On the other hand, when the composition of a food is altered unnaturally, we create non-foods that cannot be used at all. Soy-based products have flooded the market due to the perception of soy as a health food. The soy is processed with solvents, extracted into oils, broken down into defatted flours, isolated or textured or otherwise changed entirely from its original form. Soy is cheap, easily produced with the aid of Round-up, and sells well. (Samsel, Seneff, 2013) These soy products should be avoided like any other unrecognizable food product.

Dairy

Some will argue that dairy is entirely unnecessary in any circumstance. And, as we know, some public health sources advocate dairy as an absolute necessity. Yet again, the truth is probably somewhere in between. Throughout human history, the milk and fermented products (cheese, butter, buttermilk) of the herd would help to sustain the family and community. But can you spot the interference? The milk we've used for generations looks very different today.

The first interference came with pasteurization. It's a necessary step for safety when milk is going to be stored and delivered away from its original farm. But in destroying pathogens, it also denatures the healthy bacteria, fats, and proteins and breaks down the vitamins. That's why we can buy milk that's been fortified with vitamin D—it has to be added back once it's been damaged. We're attempting to restructure after creating damage.

The next is homogenization, which is a factor of marketing, not health or sanitation. Homogenization breaks up the fat particles to create a smooth product, and one that can be controlled for fat content—1%, 2%, whole milk. Do you remember that fat holds toxin concentrations? In its natural state, the fat is in clumps and globs. The cream at the top. If you consume it as-is, your body has clumps and globs to contend with, and the immune system can attack concentrated segments while metabolizing the rest. Once it's been homogenized, the entire cup of milk is a threat. It takes more work to process. Or, in the case of skim milk, if the fat is removed entirely, the ratios of fat and sugars (lactose) will be skewed—there goes your fat, and you've got a more sugary drink than you did before.

Lactose and casein intolerance aside, milk is a special consideration that begins with the production process. Raw milk from someone you know and trust is the obvious first choice and most closely model our ancestral roots. The next best choice would be a commercial operation that produces milk from cows who haven't been fed sprayed foods or injected with hormones or antibiotics. Non-homogenized milk is the next ideal, keeping the milk as close to natural composition as possible.

Even further—back to casein—some research has emerged in recent years suggesting that not all casein is the same. It is possible, for some, that milk containing A1 casein from Ayreshires, Jerseys, Brown Swiss and Holstein-Friesian cattle may be more problematic than A2 casein from Guernsey cattle, goats, and sheep. (betacasein.org, 2017) Therefore, in choosing dairy for consumption, there is no hierarchy—it's more like a checklist. Depending on where you live and where you buy your groceries, it may be difficult to check every single box on your list. Do the best that you can, and listen to your body to know what works for you and what doesn't.

Advanced Nutrition in Special Circumstances

Some of the exclusions in the Advanced Plan have been at the center of controversy, and it's important to know why we've made these considerations. For example, few will disagree that refined grains should be eliminated. But why would we include all grains? Why limit so many kinds of fruits?

First, know that an exclusion from the Advanced Plan does not mean that food is bad or unhealthy. Remember, we are working in triage mode here, taking extra care with a body that has been through a great deal. You may find that you thrive without grains, or you might work certain grains back into your diet once you're ready. For now, if you're following the Advanced Plan, you are simply taking extra precautions to accelerate health changes and, in some cases, maintain an exceptional level of well being because you know that it works for you.

Second, understand that the goal with this plan is not to reduce calories or force weight loss, as is so often the case when diets exclude grains. Instead, we are hoping to reset the body's use of fats and sugars, along with the hormone signals that those imbalances cause.

So, a complete and sudden shift away from the high-glycemic fruits and all grains removes as much sugar from the diet, all at once, as possible. Easing into this plan will not be as beneficial. Full disclosure: this is not easy and should only be undertaken when you're ready. The first two weeks can be incredibly difficult (though, it almost universally levels off after that). The sudden change takes away the source of energy and fat storage that the body has relied on and forces it to find something else—the fat it should have been burning all along. Dropping glycemic intake all at once also restructures the hormone signaling—insulin and leptin—that alters the way we balance minerals, fluids, and even hunger itself.

Give your body time to adapt to the increased fat intake so that you can efficiently digest what you eat and use it for energy. But the elimination of grains and fruits will not have the same effect in a gradual shift.

Note as well that the Advanced Plan goes grain free, not simply gluten free. Although gluten allergies and celiac disease are very real, we're looking deeper than the concept of gluten-intolerance. Conventional wheat has many strikes against it— far more than gluten alone. The Roundup-soaking method called "desiccation" is one concern. (Davis, 2012) Our bodies could simply be damaged and worn down by extensive residual toxins. But the other problem with the gluten-free craze has come in the form of marketing. Much like the sell-factor associated with low-fat, soy, or sugar-free, gluten-free has given rise to countless processed products that manufacturers know will sell simply because the term "gluten-free" is associated with health.

If you're struggling with inflammation, pain, fatigue, and illness, getting off gluten will probably make you feel better. But there's likely a bigger beast behind it, and the Advanced Plan aims to dig it out and get rid of it for good.

Beyond the Advanced Plan

The goal of the 5 Essentials is to reconnect you with your body. What is that innate wisdom telling you? If you dive into the Advanced Plan and find it needs to be adjusted—not that you're craving something sweet and want to be done, but actually *need* a change—will you listen closely enough to your body to know? There will be cases where specific illnesses or sensitivities lead you to adjust these plans to meet your needs. This is where it helps to partner with a practitioner who can guide you through these changes in diet and lifestyle.

For example, you might already require a ketogenic diet. Some people have worked with practitioners to use ketogenesis as a tool to feed their bodies in response to major illness. Though the Advanced Plan might already fall in line with keto—this would largely depend on other individualized factors; you can take it to your care provider to find a balance that works for you.

Remember that we don't pursue any of the essentials in order to force a cure. If chiropractic doesn't immediately fix a long-term illness, you don't toss your appointment book out the window. If you make the change to your nutrition plan and don't see immediate healing, you are *still* doing great things for your body— keep at it! Some people allow their bodies to heal, even in unseen ways, for short-term trials on the Advanced Plan. Others find they enjoy it indefinitely. You can only try. **Gift your body these good foods and let it heal as it will.**

Your individualized needs will shift and vary based on your genetics, your life to this point, what's feasible, what's necessary, and what should be prioritized. You might walk away with a combination or alternating version of the two plans. You might adjust it to make something entirely new. Our plans are baseline guides formulated after years of study and work with countless clients. Use them to bring your body back to that innate knowledge—to use food as intended and to fuel your journey through the 5 Essentials.

Breaking from Old Rules

Shira Krieger

Going into a MaxLiving workshop as a cardiac nurse, I knew in advance that much of what I would learn was going to be the opposite of what nursing school had taught me.

But, several years ago, I had reached my heaviest weight— and I had to do something. I had been basing my food choices on the heart-healthy diet I learned about in nursing school. I was overweight and struggled with low energy levels, so I was willing to give what I was learning about the 5 Essentials a shot. Plus, the workshop came at a perfect time,

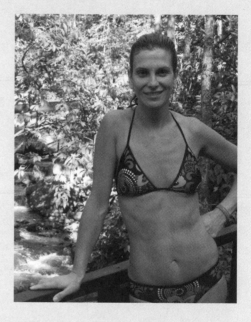

right after Christmas when I stepped on the scales and felt disgusted with myself for eating so terribly over the holidays.

To be honest, MaxLiving's wholesome, organic, clean, toxin-free approach initially terrified me! I felt like I was an awful mother, feeding what I thought were healthy foods to my children. It was no wonder we had so many health issues.

I also sat there learning about fats and sugars and remember thinking, "What am I supposed to tell my patients?"... It was the opposite of what I had always learned.

But that MaxLiving workshop would change everything.

I started out with small steps, changing only my diet initially, and gradually implementing those healthy changes into my family's life. Knowing that I needed to make some quick changes, and that I had consumed a lot of toxic food in my history, I followed the Advanced Plan initially. I knew that taking the more dramatic approach would yield better results than just slowly easing up on what I ate. That hadn't worked for me in the past.

I set a goal to lose thirty to thirty-five pounds, which I thought was reasonable. To my surprise, my weight fell off like never before. It almost felt effortless because I was eating so much good food and yet consistently losing weight.

I have exceeded those goals ... I've lost fifty-two pounds! I feel so much better. I have more energy at work, more mental clarity, and more confidence.

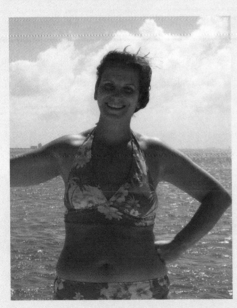

BEFORE

When I did a follow-up checkup, my doctor praised my blood work. He was a little concerned about the amount of dietary fat I was eating and what that might do to my cholesterol and lipid profile—but all those numbers came out perfect.

I've lost all this weight without doing much exercise at all. Exercise is what I'm focusing on next. My bigger-picture goals include teaching my family and young kids to develop better eating habits. At this point, it's not about weight loss. It's about experiencing great health.

CHAPTER 5

Innate Movement

The 5 Essentials are not meant to be stacked up in a hierarchy or checked off like a to-do list. Altogether, they are a way of life that combine for maximized health. Individually, focusing on any one of them can help to eliminate another piece of interference that might be holding you back, body and mind. Exercise and oxygen are paired together as one essential, because this is not just for aspiring athletes. It's not a call to sell your life to a gym. It's not about body shape or size. The essential need here is to move your body as it was intended so that it can function as intended.

That said, if you are a recreational athlete, or even a competitive or aspiring athlete, the principles of MaxLiving can help you reach even higher goals in your athletic quest. When you bring the body back to its ideal state, you can ward off injuries, promote healing and repair, and—a major concern for anyone whose career depends on athleticism—longevity.

Exercise and Oxygen

Exercise, first and foremost, helps your heart and lungs to move oxygen and nutrients through the body. We can free the nervous system with chiropractic care, and we can feed our bodies good, nutritious foods—but without regular exercise, none of those good things will make it to our cells, tissues, muscles and organs. Exercise is vital, not only for the more visible muscles in your arms and legs and core, but for your lungs and heart. **It very well may be that you're body's number one missing nutrient is oxygen.**

Because the 5 Essentials are about making realistic, effective changes, it has to be the *right kind* of exercise. Your body was designed to move. Not necessarily to scale mountains or run marathons—though these things can certainly be achieved—but to stretch, walk, lift, squat, carry, press, and move. Modern lifestyles take us from bed to car to office to couch. Moving has become the exception rather than the norm, and we're paying for it not only with our health but our lives. In October 2017, an internal medicine journal reported that a highly sedentary lifestyle can be a risk factor for all-cause mortality. (Diaz, et al, 2017) In other words: **Sitting is taking years off of your life.**

Being athletic or running marathons won't make you younger—even if it does lengthen your life (and that's debatable)—but that might not be a goal for you anyway. As we'll see, *prolonged cardio isn't the most biologically natural goal.* The MaxLiving life is about bringing your body as close to its intended purpose and function as possible, and no traditional or ancestral society ran great distances on paved surfaces.

Instead, the MaxLiving approach is to look for ways to condition our bodies to high bursts of energy within a lifestyle of consistent movement. With this essential focus, you'll help your body become accustomed to exercise and develop a strong cardiovascular system, bringing oxygen and nutrients to all parts of the body.

Our goal is to work *with* the body's design rather than *against* it. We aren't panda bears, sitting back on our tails and eating all day long. We aren't gazelles, upright and running great distances. The human body is versatile and strong, designed to squat, crawl, climb, push, pull, and move around our environments in powerful ways throughout the day. And ignoring the body's design carries heavy consequences, whether you realize it or not.

An Ancestry of Movement

Intentional exercise is a relatively new phenomenon. For most of human history, there was no need to work out. As recently as pre-Industrial Revolution, the daily rigors of life required us to be active and fit. It wasn't until automation brought workers in to stand at machines and corporate leaders to sit behind desks that we all stopped moving. Now, it's more common than not to sit behind a desk, in a car, at a kitchen table, or in front of the television.

Sit, sit, sit.

Ancestral lives were always in motion. Think back to campfires and hunter/gatherers. Bending, squatting, crawling, reaching, and sprinting had to be normal functions of life. Adrenaline and cortisol would spike to provide energy and protect the body during dangerous situations like hunting or defense, then the body would resume normal function in times of calm and fasting. Stress responses ebbed and flowed, protecting the body and mind.

The posture that a chair requires would have been foreign to anyone in our early history. Each of those innate movements created balance and core strength, while fostering loose limbs and responsive cardiovascular health. All of the things we aspire to in a session at the gym or a practice of meditation would have come as a natural course of life.

In so many ways, *sitting* in our modern era has become the new smoking.

That's not hyperbole. In fact, not even time in the gym can reverse the effects of a lifestyle of sitting. Excessive screen time has been linked to a nearly 50% increase in death from any cause and 125% increase of cardiovascular problems, yes, but any form of extended sitting can be dangerous. Desks, TV time, and car time are all logged the same when it comes to health risks. (Levine, 2015)

Researchers have been exploring posture concerns for decades. A cursory look at research shows stacks of papers concerned with chair posture, work posture, school posture. In the '80s, researchers questioned why tables and chairs were designed so that it's impossible to work and read without hunching over your materials. (Mandal, 1986) Well over thirty years later, our tables and chairs look largely the same.

As we discussed in chapter 3, posture is vital for spine health. But it takes more than just an aligned spine to hold good posture. All of the muscles anchored to the spine—neck, shoulders, core, even buttocks—support the body as you stand and sit upright. Hunching shoulders and a slouching, passive seated position can weaken those muscles, and so can a lack of exercise. When you're hunched over and folded into yourself, from the slightest to the most dramatic of posture concerns, your nervous system is compromised, your organs are pressed, and your circulatory system is slowed—and sometimes blocked.

As you begin work on this essential, picture your body working as it was meant to. Think about the deep breaths that will carry oxygen deep into your lungs, fueling the blood that wraps around all of your organs and flows in and out of all of your cells. Imagine the obstacles that oxygen might face when you're hunched over, slouching, and sitting. Be aware of these movements throughout the day, because a MaxLiving life isn't reserved for the gym. Every step that we take toward whole-body health is a step toward a lifestyle of constant awareness. We're not exercising to meet a goal. A lifestyle of movement *is* the goal.

Short Surges of Energy

The body makes no distinction between a bear attack, a big meeting with the CEO, or even intense and prolonged cardio. That's because stress itself is simply a threat to homeostasis—the body's mechanisms that keep everything in balance. All of the mechanisms that respond to stress are meant to protect short-term threats.

For many of us, adopting an intense, prolonged cardio routine is nothing more than an added stress. Our joints and tendons protest, it's frustrating to fit it into the schedule, and the shift toward intense, prolonged exercise can trigger internal stress response.

The goal of MaxLiving exercise is to re-train the body to respond to short bursts of physical stress and then return to normal. Together with the maximized mind, we're restructuring the stress response and, in turn, releasing a cascade of health benefits.

The surge principle accomplishes this goal effectively, by building up both strength and endurance without prolonging physical stress. The idea is to move as powerfully as possible for short amounts of time, then rest. As a principle, this can be applied to any form of exercise at any skill level. Sprinting, weight lifting, swimming, resistance and body weight exercises—any kind of movement can be adapted to a surge principle.

As an added benefit, you can pack much more effort and return into small amounts of time. No one expects you to find an hour or more in your schedule. High Impact Intensity Training (HIIT) exercises that we often utilize and recommend are quick and much easier to work into a normal day than long hours on the treadmill or running in the elements.

As with all exercise plans—but especially with high intensity work—be smart and safe as you implement any kind of surge exercises. Ease into them from wherever your skill level is now, building strength and resilience over time.

Remember that muscle soreness is different than muscle pain: heed the warnings. Check with your doctor to make sure you don't have any precluding conditions, and check with your chiropractor to make sure you don't have any injuries or issues that require adaptation of the exercises. The goal is always to listen to our bodies and what they need, and it's more important here than ever!

Building Strength

In 2016, researchers zeroed in on a potential protective treatment for the gut permeability that comes with heavy exercise. They found some success, but that's not the intriguing thing. What's interesting is the premise: *heavy exercise leads to gut issues, even permeability.* So if we keep a sedentary lifestyle, our bodies are at risk. But if we swing toward the opposite and run our bodies through the wringer, our immune systems, hormones, and even our gut health will be at risk. We're doing something wrong.

In the middle, we find a lifestyle of movement coupled with HIIT exercises following the burst principle. Building strength through surges of big movement avoids the damage that prolonged, heavy exercise can do. When you use your body weight as resistance, you can build that strength organically—fewer supplies to buy and less damage done to your adapting body.

Lower body strength will come naturally with the steps and bursts of any of the movements. Upper body strength can be built simply by lifting your arms during the bursts—with or without weights, depending on where you're starting—pressing against door frames or doing push-ups against the wall, or including whole-body movements like swimming.

You'll also find that creating a life in motion—a standing desk, regular walks, stretching and flexing during periods of sitting, using good posture—will build the muscles that keep you moving. Strength doesn't have to come from a gym. For most of us, simply engaging our muscles throughout the day will tone and build strength. In the appendix, you'll find some examples of regular exercises that you can incorporate into your routine. For now, let's look at the concept of the surge cycle.

A Boost of Better Cardio

To this point, it sounds like we could build the case that cardio can be forgotten forever. Don't misunderstand: surge training will absolutely work and improve your cardiovascular health. It's not a complete loss of cardio—it's a better, more efficient kind of cardio. When untrained, middle-aged men were placed on a 16-week exercise program, those working on a running program lost fat, but they also lost muscle alongside it. By contrast, the group who practiced a HIIT program had better cardio-metabolic results and skipped the muscle loss. (Kemmler, et al, 2015)

That's what we're going for here. Quick bursts of cardio and muscular effort, without extending it into fatigue and an unfavorable hormone, immune, and muscle-loss response.

In practical terms, the research supports a burst of energy that gets your heart rate up, followed by a period of recovery, repeated two or three times before taking a longer rest at your lower heart rate.

You might recognize the principle as Tabata, HIIT, or interval training, but you can modify it to almost any exercise and skill level. An elite athlete might be able to sprint with full exertion for a full minute, but then a break for 3-4 minutes would be warranted. Beginners might stick closer to 20 seconds on, 20 seconds off, then 10 seconds off as endurance builds, then longer intervals when you're ready. Intensity can vary, too—30 percent intensity on one cycle, then 40 percent, ramping up as you go.

As you build your endurance, you'll be able to repeat the cycle repeated times, then spend the rest of your day focusing on posture and active life choices.

There is plenty of room for customization with the concept of surge training, as long as you stick to the shorter intervals with some rests in between. We want to stretch the capacity of the heart, lungs, and muscles, without becoming a source of stress and extensive fatigue.

If you aren't sure where to begin, we find that 20 seconds on and 20 seconds off for a total of 12 minutes of exertion is not only achievable for all athletic types, but it gets great results. The customization is almost limitless.

Sprint, cycle, rollerblade, swim, step, walk, play—what is it that you'd *like* to do? Do it in bursts with time to recover. As you improve your cardio health and muscular strength and want to scale up the bursts, add weights, intensity or reps rather than time in the burst. Don't extend these high-intensity moments so far that the stress response is triggered or injuries are risked. As with anything else in the body, once there is pain, injury, or disease, much more invisible damage will have already been done.

These cardio bursts aren't just great for circulation—they also affect hormone optimization. Hormones, as we know, control fat burning and stimulate muscle growth. Bulking aside, if you're surging sprints, you don't necessarily have to add bicep curls to have great arms. This is notably in opposition to distance running, which typically wastes muscle away in order to provide the energy it requires.

Flexibility

A key part of the active lifestyle you'll want to build in between burst sessions is flexibility. Can you still touch your toes? Can you stretch your arms up and bend to each side or arch your back? If you were to sit on the floor, how long would it take you to get back up to standing? Not only are these questions of mobility, but they underscore the strength and flexibility required to support a healthy spine.

When was the last time you tried to get up from a seated position on the floor? Did you have to roll over, get on all fours, then ease your way up? The ability to sit down on the floor and get back up *without using your hands* can tell you a lot about your flexibility, posture, and muscle strength, which tells you even more about your health at any age. One group of men over fifty took this test, and then researchers followed up with all of them several years later to find that the less likely they were to perform this sit/rise test, the higher the mortality rates. (Brito, et al, 2014) We often take creaking joints and a ten-step standing-up system for granted, especially as we age. This doesn't have to be the case. Flexibility, posture, and strength are important to pursue and maintain from childhood to the twilight of life.

Flexibility will naturally improve with better posture, as will balance. But both of them can be improved with the flowing, centering movements of traditional movement practices like Tai Chi, Qi Gong, and Yoga. Adding a meditative flexibility and balance program to your regular routine is an excellent option for both exercise and oxygen intake.

There is a reason these practices have been passed down through the centuries. Long before the Greek gymnasiums—wrestling and racing, competing as Olympians, and a general obsession with physical fitness—exercise was being prescribed in Chinese and Ayurvedic medicine. Susruta, the first physician known to recommend exercise, encouraged activities that would cause fatigue and labored breathing, but only to half capacity, not over-extended. (Tipton, 2008) Chinese medicine focused on breath as well, intended to cleanse the body by creating heavier breathing. The idea was to balance exertion with breath and flexibility.

Alongside the cardio and strength rigors of daily life, a focus on stretching and cleansing breath have, from what we can see, always been recommended and practiced. Adding a meditative flexibility and balance program to your regular routine is an excellent option for both sides of the exercise and oxygen essential.

Arms up, arms down, roll your neck, touch your toes—we all have certain go-to stretches that hit the obvious muscle groups. But the arms are not separate from the legs, the shoulders aren't separate from the hips. Our bodies are single organisms, and it's important to balance the whole body, head to toe, with a full body stretch every single day.

Eating and Exercise

Pre-workout. Mid-workout fuel. Recovery. There's a bar, shake, snack, recipe, tip, trick, and trap for every single phase of an exercise routine. It's not surprising. We're all looking for that formula that will get us healthy, and big fitness industry figureheads are looking to make a buck. Meanwhile, the average person just looking to get active and feel better can get caught up in a lot of confusion and unnecessary products.

At some point in a health or fitness journey, most of us have been or will be obsessed with what they are eating in every waking moment. That's no way to live. And it's no way to develop a healthy relationship with our bodies and food, either.

In fact, maybe our bodies just need a defined rest from all that caring and all that eating. We're not talking about going days without food, but there is something to allowing your body prolonged rests from eating. Ramadan participants, in a 2012 study, had lower inflammation scores during their holiday that requires no eating at all until the sun goes down. (Faris, et al, 2012)

Whatever the cause of improvement, we know it certainly wasn't a patented food product or newly developed supplement that did the trick. You shouldn't have to hunt down those products for your workout, either. Good food is good food, and the Core or Advanced Nutrition Plans have loads of foods that you can choose for any meal, no matter when your burst training is scheduled.

In fact, there is merit to planning your workout first thing in the morning, near the end of the "fast" we all participate in daily: the break in eating between the time you fall asleep and the time you *break-fast* in the morning.

Both stress and perceived starvation trigger protective hormone responses. When utilized intentionally, these processes can be used to our advantage—starvation, of course, being a simple break in mealtimes. Insulin, hunger cues, and metabolism are among the processes regulated in times of intermittent—but not prolonged to the point of deprivation—fasting.

For example, growth hormone actually increases in times of fasting—potentially to make up for the growth that nutrition would otherwise trigger. (Ho, et al, 1988) Intermittent fasting, or exercising on an empty stomach before breakfast, could take advantage of that growth hormone burst that helps with muscle recovery.

Intermittent fasting was the subject of a 2009 study comparing weight loss during normal diet and exercise with a routine of modified fasting. (Varady, et al, 2009) The results validated intermittent fasting as a viable strategy for weight loss. What's more, one study monitored the way the body might source its fuel when exercising on an empty stomach. They found that intramyocellular triglycerides—a contributor to diabetes—was burned off during the exercise. (Loon, et al, 2003)

Of course, any heart, weight, or hormonal benefits are nullified if you're stressed out, either consciously agitated by the skipped meal or unconsciously taxing a body that needs to eat. A healthy, working intermittent fast would look like a consistent choice to postpone the morning meal or skip a meal in the evening. It would be bolstered by excellent meal choices throughout the day and prioritized sleep at night. You have to get all of the food you need, from good sources, in fewer meals, which takes a concerted effort. This is *not* dieting or calorie restriction.

What's more—most of these studies have focused on men, not women, and that's an important distinction to make. Hormones run differently between the genders, and homeostasis protecting reproductive systems and menstrual cycles create different functions in the body. This could also trace back to ancestral patterns, since what we know of that era tells us women more often stayed out of the hunt and instead protected children and the camp. We've seen men thrive on intermittent fasting while women might see changes in their cycle and general malaise. On the other hand, a 2012 study noted intermittent fasting could benefit women in weight loss, even reducing risks of heart disease. (Klempel, et al, 2012)

These mixed conclusions take us back to the original premise: eating and exercise don't have to be complicated. Frankly, for a multitude of reasons, some individuals may just feel and function better on a fuller stomach. You know your body best, and you can tell when something is helping you to thrive or when you feel depleted and ill.

Women, if you've been intermittently fasting or exercising on an empty stomach and your hormones seem out of balance—changes to menstrual cycles, low energy, hair loss, mood instability, too much weight loss or gain, dizziness—stop. Men, if you're not thriving, stop. Make good food choices, keep moving throughout the day, train your body with bursts of energy, and don't stress the details. No shake, bar, product, or even fasting will be the *right* answer. **All you really need to do is eat well and keep moving.**

Common Questions

We realize that our society is dominated by detailed plans, strict rules, and step-by-step "tricks" to getting exercise just right. Stepping back to such a simplified plan can be just as confusing as a program with a dozen steps and twice as many rules. It can help to work with your chiropractor, especially one trained in MaxLiving principles, to help ease your mind and walk alongside you in this journey. But we can also answer a few of the most common questions here, as well.

Do you really need protein right after your workout?

Outside of basic RDA, there's little agreement on the exact amount of protein certain body types, situations, and activity levels require in a given day. One thing's for sure: people selling protein powders want you to have *a lot*. When it comes to exercise specifically, it's important to know why you'd need that (or any) protein before determining when or how much.

The body doesn't manufacture energy from thin air any more than a car can drive without a fuel source. Something has to be used up—burned, as we so often say—in order to keep powering through the activity. Athletes sometimes stock up on carbohydrates before a big endurance event to provide energy (more on that in just a moment), and replenish with protein afterward. The thought is that the carbohydrates provide initial fuel, while muscles will be broken down for the rest of it, then protein must be required to rebuild and repair those muscles.

Though not everyone is running long distances, protein and fat stores are still broken into for energy when exercising, and if your goal is to build muscle, you'll definitely want to supply the body with enough protein in order to account for both the loss and the intended gains.

Now, whether that protein needs to be obtained immediately after a workout is up for some debate. Traditionally treated as a given, some researchers have questioned the concept of a "magic hour" after working out. The protein you eat at meals surrounding your workout will still be there, ready and working, after you've exercised. (Aragon, Schoenfeld, 2013)

The key, then, is to consider basic recommended amounts of protein, then adapt for your body type, activity level, and the type of intentional exercise you're doing. If you feel like you aren't thriving on your exercise routine, try adjusting the protein levels in your meals first.

Depending on the type and amount of exercise you are doing, you certainly need to ensure that your body's protein synthesis keeps up with your body's protein breakdown. This is where good meal planning and the occasional protein supplement can be of benefit.

Can you follow the Advanced Plan and still do distance cardio?

Running isn't the worst thing in the world. In 2012, researchers said that running decreases mortality by 19%—that is, until distances are factored in. *Too much running* does start to bump the risks back up again. Under 20 miles per week was the sweet spot for benefits without added stress.

The disconnect between running and the Advanced Plan appears to happen in carbs. If you're running distances, you'll need some carbs to fuel your run, so how does that work when we're limiting so many of the go-to sources? The answer is in just that: *the sources.*

Even the most restrictive forms of ketogenic diets leave room for some carbohydrate intake. (Pendergast, 2013) We need a balance of macronutrients, even though the ratios that create balance might differ from person to person. My father—by way of anecdote—was an exceptional marathon runner. He ran at the fastest times for his age group when he was sixty years old. The day before a marathon, he'd eat a single bowl of pasta. Other than that, he trained without increased carbs.

Now, I watched him run for three hours straight on a high fat, high protein diet plus one weekly bowl of pasta, so I have little trouble believing that other nutrients are important for endurance athletes and no qualms at all for the rest of us.

Keep your macros balanced as necessary for your body. When you're training, you can adapt the Advanced Plan to your needs. If you need to go for high-sugar/low-fiber carbs before your run, that's fine. But it's simply not necessary as a regular practice.

What if I want to gain weight?

In a society of obesity, people struggling with issues of low weight are often overlooked. All too often, health is associated with looking trim, but sometimes being thin can be as much of a reflection of an unhealthy body as being overweight. We don't want to miss you in these discussions!

Low weight might be as simple as genetics and a naturally fast metabolism, or it could reflect complex illnesses of the thyroid, gut, autoimmune disease, endocrine system, or neurological complication. There might be problems with hyperthyroidism, small intestinal bacterial overgrowth (SIBO), intestinal permeability, type 1 diabetes, or other chronic or autoimmune disease, neurological disease, or more.

Usually, when someone brings up this concern, those conditions wind up in the minority. If you're struggling with low weight, the first step you need to take is to be checked out by your physician. When you've been given the all clear, revisit your motivation. Maybe your diet has been too lean for too long, and the weight loss has moved beyond healthy proportions.

As discussed in chapter 4, the Advanced Plan might work long term for some people, while others only need it for a short amount of time. Above all, however, remember that the Advanced Plan is not about caloric restriction—it's designed to help re-establish normal hormone balance in the body. I do believe that is why I've worked with countless individuals looking to put on healthy weight, and they've done so by using the Advanced Plan exclusively. **It's all about reaching your body's innately-driven, optimal shape and size.** Try it, first!

Then, if you wish to take it a bit further, or perhaps even bulk up a bit, consider opening your diet up to some of the real foods found in the basic, Core Nutrition Plan in order to stack some starches and varied nutrients into your diet again. You can still watch the *way* you consume them—eating starches at night or without your regular exercise routine will only stack fat, not healthy weight. But starchy foods in the form of real-food, complex carb sources might help you stabilize your weight and feel better doing it.

If you haven't been eating well—or if crash dieting has sent you spiraling—the Advanced Plan can first address any damage from dieting or hormonal stress, then the slow additions of good starches can up the calories while protecting that innate health. This can look like a baked sweet potato hash for breakfast, whole grain rice added to your lunch, or any of the healthy, complex carbs included on the Core Plan listed in the back of the book. Incorporate them at or before lunch, giving your body from the afternoon on to adapt and process them fully.

Healthy, protein-rich smoothies are another great way to add nutrients. Grind nuts like almonds or cashews before adding the rest of your smoothie ingredients, or add a bit of avocado for a creamy texture and added fats. Changing up the types of fruits in the smoothie can increase carb intake without losing focus. Fresh or frozen bananas are a smoothie favorite and just above the sugar levels recommended when you're on the Advanced Plan. As you adapt your diet to gain weight, continue to source your foods well, add foods with care, and enjoy the higher carb content early in the day. But, remember: the worst carb you'll ever consume is the one your body doesn't utilize. Therefore, up your carbs only when you're exerting more through exercise. And even then, some genetic types may not need to.

Note: *Any "protein packing" (more than what your body needs in relation to your activity level) can begin to risk the balance of health we're hoping to achieve. You can only process so much protein or work your muscles so far before it becomes a stress in itself. Lifting heavy weights is the only way to build muscle, and protein should be used to supplement—not to enhance or spike muscle building into overdrive.*

Focus on the essentials, make sure you don't have any underlying health issues, and give your body time to develop in a whole and complete way.

Starting on a Better Path

Linda Ziglar

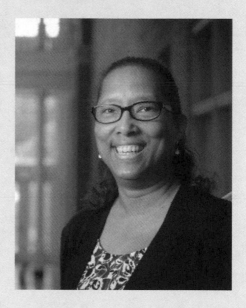

" One year ago, I was taking medication for high cholesterol, acid reflux, thyroid, plus hormone replacement therapy (HRT) and a host of others to control my allergies. I would get anywhere from three to four sinus infections every year (sometimes more), and I would contract bronchitis so badly that it would lead to pneumonia and I would be out of work for weeks. I also suffered with depression— but I refused to go on one more medication. All I could do by 5:00 pm was sit on the sofa. My energy was in the tank.

I joined my sister at a celebration dinner with others, who had in the past experienced issues similar to mine. They were sharing their stories of recovery through five essentials for health and wellbeing. The testimonials blew me away, but I was skeptical. I had been struggling for over twenty years with my health challenges. But I committed to a lifestyle change with MaxLiving. I got connected with the chiropractor, started taking better care of my spine and body, changed my nutrition, and started on a better path with those 5 Essentials. I loved the workouts because most exercise is otherwise boring to me. I got started with high intensity workouts at home, burst running, and even took my regimen to work, making a point of doing ten-minute intervals up and down the flights up stairs.

One of the first things I noticed was that my energy level went through the roof! It was amazing—the best energy I had felt in years! **Before I knew it, I could keep up with my four-year-old grandson, and spend more time with my husband outdoors.**

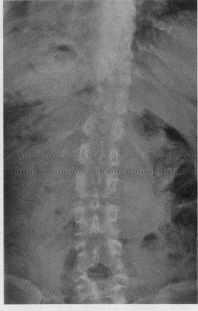 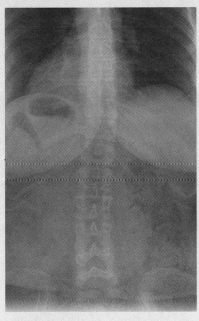

BEFORE   AFTER

Throughout the process of care, not only did Linda's lab values improve; her lumbar curvature was reduced from 9° to 5°.

I've not experienced any mood or depression symptoms. My hormones are more stable. I've lost over twenty pounds. I'm no longer taking any medications for cholesterol, acid reflux or my thyroid, and I've also been able to discontinue HRT without any issues. With good nutrition, my allergies are almost nonexistent.

When my doctor noticed my diminishing need for medication, she asked me what I was doing. I told her about MaxLiving. Her comment to me was, "Keep doing what you're doing."

I love my life now, feeling good every day.

CHAPTER 6

Freeing the Body of Toxins

Your body was designed for health. Its mechanisms are constantly analyzing and adjusting for balance both externally and internally. *Homeostasis*—the sense of normalcy and balance required for your body to work—is always the priority, and your organs, hormones, and nerves work in concert to communicate about what needs to change in order to preserve it. Sometimes, vital processes are preserved at the expense of how you feel.

What does all of that have to do with toxins? Everything! Trashing toxins is not just about a checklist of *good* or *bad* products and exposures. It's about minimizing the work required of your body for excess detoxification.

The priorities of homeostasis are nothing short of amazing, and they would be all we need in a pure environment. That's the innate at work. We've already seen how the stress response works well under short term, emergent threats, but can contribute to life-threatening disease in our current stress situations.

Similarly, the liver, skin, and excretory organs, even the stomach, are extremely effective detoxification systems when risk is infrequent. The inhalation of campfires, the accidental ingestion of a plant toxin—all of the incidental toxins that would have been a threat in a nomadic or agrarian life are easily removed by the body.

But in today's world, every minute of every day, we are bombarded with toxins. The chemical, toxic interference of modern life is astounding. Outdoor pollution is a problem, yes, but inside your home is even worse. We've pushed far beyond the limits of what our bodies were meant to encounter. Yet onward our organs and hormones go, sending a constant response that winds up looking like painful inflammation and autoimmune disease, or perhaps shutting off the response entirely and letting carcinogenic toxins do their work.

Our job, in this age of continual exposure, is to do the work of toxin removal before our bodies have to. **As much as possible, we've got to trash the toxins.**

Toxins vs. Toxicants

The term "toxin" has been thrown around in clickbait headlines for a long time. In response, something of a callus has formed over the word, and skeptics question whether toxins are a concern at all. So, let's back up and talk about what we mean by these terms before we keep going.

A toxin can be generalized as anything that causes disease. But our society, down to even the healthiest of homes, is inundated with so many pollutants that keeping track of the classification groups alone can be overwhelming. There are aerosols, sulfates, sulfites, and nitrites; pesticides, herbicides, and insecticides. Some affect the nerves, the lungs, the skin, the liver, or combinations of each, not to mention the environment. Then there are the varying messages about toxins that conflict with each other. How do we know what is safe, what might be dose-dependent, and are we actually in danger from so many sources?

Since we're talking about some of the smallest, often undetectable components of the products in our lives, let's break the discussion down as far as we can, as well. It's true that all matter is composed of chemicals—so *chemicals* themselves are not our concern, even though "chemical-free" is used frequently as a generalized buzzword.

It's also true, to some extent, that the dose can make the poison, so that even the healthiest substances can become toxic to our bodies if we overindulge to the point of danger. You've probably heard someone list the ails of *dihydrogen-monoxide.* Consume too much at once and it's fatal, though everyone who has ever consumed it has or will die, anyway. The "chemical" in question, of course is H_2O—water! Or you might have seen a long and complicated ingredient list that is then revealed to be the chemical composition of an apple.

The natural dangers found in venom, mushrooms, or "too much of a good thing," are considered true toxins. When we decide to minimize toxins as part of the 5 Essentials, we're looking for the toxins that are man-made, unnatural additions to our environment that the body is not prepared to process. Technically, these are *toxicants*, and they interfere with our health in pervasive and devastating ways. Unlike pathogenic bacteria and viruses, the symptoms that many of these toxins provoke are often subtle, sometimes going completely unrecognized until they have accumulated.

Out of Sight, Out of Mind

Often, when you change your diet or habits in some way and begin to feel better, it can seem like you feel bad more often. Maybe you're more sore a week after a chiropractic appointment, or a junk food you used to enjoy now makes your stomach hurt and your head feel foggy. It's not that life affects you *more* than it used to—but you didn't know how just bad you felt all the time when *feeling bad* was your sense of normal.

Toxins—actually toxicants, but for the sake of familiarity, we'll stick with "toxins"—affect the body in a similar way. **In the past few decades, more than 100,000 new chemicals have been introduced to our bodies, homes, and environment.** (Yang, 2014) Stop and let that sink in for a moment: 100,000 *brand new* things for the immune system and detoxification pathways to adapt to. New things for the environment to adjust around. And all of them introduced during the Baby Boomer, Gen X, and Millennial generations.

The 2014 study that brought us those numbers looked at the concurrent rise in allergies and asked whether the two could be connected. How often have we marveled at the prevalence of diseases that our grandparents hardly even knew? Allergies, asthma, cancer, cognitive and mood disorders, inflammatory disease— all on the rise over the past few decades. In the review on allergies alone, the authors cite links between allergies and phthalates, tobacco smoke, heavy metals, diesel exhaust, particulate matter (debris), and pesticides. The American Cancer Society lists dozens of known carcinogens—from workplace exposures to food products—that are not only approved but are part of everyday life for millions of people. (cancer.org, 2017) Another review names food, polluted waters, and air itself as sources of lead, mercury, arsenic, and cadmium heavy metal exposure, connected with neurotoxic effects, cancers, and more. (Järup, 2003)

So when we say that toxins are everywhere, it's nowhere near hyperbole. Even more insidious, their effects are often silent. As a society, we're growing accustomed to things like allergies and inflammation as a matter of course. Everyone knows someone who has had cancer, or you will know someone who does, eventually. All too often, we accept them as unfortunate things that just seem to happen. Meanwhile, candies loaded with artificial colors and flavors and tons of body-weakening sugar are "pink-washed" and sold to us in the name of cancer awareness.

Silent or obvious, toxicants and toxins alike start to accumulate from the time a baby is in their mother's womb and continue throughout their lives. In 2009, the Environmental Working Group published findings of BPA (among other toxicants) in fetal cord blood—meaning the mothers had been exposed, it crossed the placental barrier, and made it into the umbilical cord. (EWG, 2009) They won't often be considered a cause of death, nor will they improve quality of life. But by doing everything you can to trash the toxins that have invaded your life and your body, you have nothing to lose and everything to gain.

But I Turned Out Fine—I Think.

Have you ever heard someone say, "I did all of those things for all my life, and I'm doing just fine!"—only to wonder what their definition of "fine" is? They might have arthritis, digestive issues, and a high risk of cancer, but because they blend right in with the millions of other people with the same laundry list of conditions, they assume this is as good as it gets. Because we aren't experiencing immediate, dramatic symptoms of toxicity—like food poisoning or a chemical burn—we figure we're doing alright. Little bits can't hurt, right? Unfortunately, nothing could be further from the truth.

When presented with a large dose of a toxin or threatening substance, the body tends to react quickly and violently. Vomiting, fever, shaking, pain and inflammation at topical contact—the big reactions let us know we've come in contact with something horrible and, assuming survival, we should never do that thing again! But smaller traces don't warrant that reaction, and they don't leave us with that important lesson.

So while the immune system might be working overtime to clear the body of trace particles of toxins—or the liver could be wearing down in its effort to clean the blood as it carries the load of more and more toxic substances—the rest of the body is largely unengaged and certainly not violently expelling anything. We often have no idea that something is wrong until we're diagnosed with the dis-ease, and even then it's difficult to know exactly what caused it.

To bring this into perspective, consider a food sensitivity compared with a food allergy, or a gluten sensitivity vs Celiac disease. Someone with a food or gluten sensitivity has a legitimate problem with that food. Their body won't break the food down properly, and at some point there will be negative consequences. But they are often symptoms that we confuse with other things, like a stomach ache, inflammation, or congestion. Unless you're looking for it, you might not know it's there. Meanwhile, a food intolerance or a gluten intolerance at the level of Celiac disease usually makes itself known in ways that are difficult to miss.

In a similar way, traces of toxic substances might not present with a violent reaction, but the damage is not any less real.

Consider the fetal connection to maternal toxin exposure that we just discussed. We're clearly becoming exposed from the earliest stages of life, well before any defense mechanisms are developed. Researchers studying the obesogenic hypothesis have documented various ways in which babies exposed to toxins like organochlorides and PDBEs have gone on to harbor extra weight, not only in animal studies but in at least one study where they followed up with studied children as adults. The weight gain usually appears later in life, and it can be difficult or impossible to overcome. (Merrell, et al, 2012)

Health at Risk

It's one thing to say we understand that toxins are bad for us. It's quite another to wrap our heads around just how much of a risk they present. In the back of the book, you'll find easy swap lists for each of these categories of risks. The problem of environmental toxins is vast, but there are practical things you can do to protect your family.

Endocrine-disruptors affect hormone signals, which are some of the most basic functions that dictate how the body should operate. Pesticides poison the air and stay as residue on food, damaging the digestive system and introducing carcinogens. These are the more well-known toxins and risks, which we'll look at more closely in a moment. First, we have to consider the risks that are hidden even deeper, often completely unacknowledged, while wreaking havoc on body and mind.

Workplace exposures are among the most dangerous, because employment is a major priority in nearly everyone's life. The workplace environment might be taken for granted as a necessary evil, or could be completely unnoticed as a health risk. Yet very real damage can be done, as the majority of a full-time employee's day is spent in an environment outside of their control.

In 2015, researchers collected data from three hundred men who had been evaluated for infertility concerns. (Wijesekara, et al, 2015) Just over half of the men had been exposed to toxins, often from their source of employment. Compared with those who had not been exposed to toxins, every single one of the sperm parameters (motility, viability, and sperm count) was lower in the group of toxin-exposed men. All of them!

In another review of occupational risks, researchers pored over what data they could regarding various workplace toxins and possible correlation with autoimmune disorders. (Cooper, et al, 2002) They note silica, solvents, pesticides, and UV radiation as the specific risks evaluated. Silica dust showed the strongest connection, increasing relative risks of rheumatoid arthritis, lupus, scleroderma, and kidney disease.

We also tend to overlook the health conditions that wouldn't seem directly connected to toxins. It's easy enough to accept that the lungs might suffer from inhaled toxins, the immune system could malfunction after bombardment, or that the digestive system would break down in response to contaminated foods. But in carefully analyzing the results of a five-year long survey (from 1999-2004), researchers found that higher levels of lead in the blood created higher risks of major depressive disorder and panic disorder in young adults. (Bouchard, et al, 2009) This supports the evidence of behavioral problems in children who have been exposed to even low levels of lead.

If we aren't concerned enough for our own health as adults, these findings should concern us for the next generation. As we've already seen, toxins accumulate in the body, then make it into a mother's breast milk and an infant's cord blood, and there are real consequences. In an assessment of over 200 infants, cognitive and psychomotor function was more likely to be delayed at a year when the cord and maternal blood had higher levels of mercury—and, like the lead studies, "higher" levels were still trace amounts. (Jedrychowski, et al, 2006) It simply does not take much—especially in light of how many different sources of exposure we're up against—to wear the body down and interfere with health.

Isolating the Sources

Be careful not to give into overwhelm here. Stress and worry are our enemies, even when they are well-intended. It's true that toxins are everywhere and that they pose great dangers, but unless you have a way to isolate yourself in a pure, natural environment, eliminating them all will be essentially impossible. **Instead, identify realistic improvements that will lighten the toxic load that your body is currently carrying.**

Food

Food is often the first point of attack for a war against toxins, and for good reason. In most cases, we have a good amount of control over the foods we purchase and eat. It's important to know right away that organic food is not completely foolproof. At least one study found some chemical residue on organic foods. (Winter, 2012) Given the alternative, however, we can be relatively confident in the choice to eat locally-sourced, organic produce whenever possible.

The first, easiest, and most economical change to make is to avoid artificial foods, colorings, and preservatives as much as possible. While toxins might be present in food in a natural state, toxicants are almost a guarantee in packaged food products. A 2002 review of food contaminants covers the various risks at each step of food processing and packaging: **The longer a food has to travel, and the more packaging involved, the greater the risk.** Industrial contaminants and byproducts from processing have to be considered alongside the pesticides and heavy metals that can be expected. (Peshin, 2002) Toxins can be transferred from metal cans, injected as emulsifiers or preservatives, and even leftover as residue from solvents used in processes like decaffeination. Remember, these processes are relatively well-regulated—this is the version of food production that is "trying" to keep us safe!

After avoiding processed and packaged foods, as well as skipping the artificial colors, flavors, and additives, you'll be left with a lot of delicious whole foods. Produce and homemade meals will rule your diet, and for awhile, you'll feel a lot better. But the next step of food-borne toxicants will be waiting for you.

The use of pesticides and herbicides might have subsided in the broad-based applications that *Silent Spring* warned against, but it's gotten more targeted. Some crops have been genetically-modified to resist pesticides, so that sprays can douse the entire plant in simpler applications without damaging the crop. Genetically-modified soybeans not only have high residues of glyphosate, but also stand out as less nutritious than organic and even conventionally-grown soybeans. (Bøhn, 2014) Organic foods are the most nutritious, and it's more than worth the effort and cost to switch to them.

By purchasing organic foods, we're also protecting workers and supporting farmers who are swimming against the tide of conventional and GM farming. Workers in farms that use pesticides, herbicides, and fungicides are at higher risk of disease, usually from direct exposure. (McCauley, et al, 2006) One review encourages organic food purchases, telling us that chronic exposure to pesticides on farms can make workers "gradually ill over a period of months or years ... when the toxic substance either accumulates in body tissues or causes minor irreversible damage at each exposure." (Kumar, et al, 2012) Memory problems, depression and mood problems, headaches, and insomnia are among the many listed consequences for conventional farmers.

Water

It's not just food at risk. Water quality can vary dramatically from source to source. Traces of contamination are the rule rather than the exception. Most municipalities will release a regular statement of water testing results. They will tell you what metals, chemicals, and general toxins were left behind in the water and to what extent, usually declaring certain amounts of chemicals to be be present but passable by EPA standards. (EPA, 2017) If your water is sourced from a well, you might not know unless you had it extensively tested yourself.

Private water systems aren't required to release these test results, either, a concern raised in 2015, when drinking water in a private system in Virginia was found to have more than the "acceptable" levels of lead in almost 20% of the cases thanks to pipe corrosion. (Pieper, 2015) Of course, even when it's a public system—as we've so tragically watched unfold in Flint, MI—clean water systems are simply not guaranteed.

The allowable levels are another concern entirely—the natural health world has watched these tragedies unfold, balked at the lists of chemicals in tap water nationwide, and questioned the wisdom in entire populations drinking toxins all day, every day. We are certainly grateful for the sanitation systems that keep us safe from microorganism contamination, but the trade-off seems to be remnants of those systems in our drinking glasses—not to mention the metals leaching from pipes, medications seeping through filtration systems, and intentional additions such as fluoride added to the process.

As part of the service of sanitation, public health determinants have decided that these things are acceptable in small levels. But that doesn't make them ideal or even safe, and it doesn't mean that we can turn a blind eye simply because they have been allowed.

Ideally, drinking water would come fresh from springs, carrying a few minerals and little else. Distilled water is another good option—though it lacks minerals, it should also lack toxins. However, any water that's been stored in a plastic bottle could have leached endocrine-disrupting phthalates, even when they are BPA-free, leading to more health concerns. (Bittner, et al, 2014) A filter for your home water can help to make your water as clean as possible. If you can't completely eliminate the risks, do what you can to eliminate the worst of them. Petrochemicals, PCBs, pharmaceutical residues, and heavy metals are at the top of the list. Forget "approved maximums," and aim for as close to zero as you can. **These small accumulations lead to big problems.**

Personal Care Products

The largest organ in the human body isn't *in* it at all, but *on* it. Your skin is your very first protection against many toxic encounters, meant to filter out what should be absorbed and what can be eliminated. And yet, personal care products meant to be slathered, soaked, and spritzed onto the skin every day are filled with manufactured ingredients. If it goes on your skin, it's safest to assume that at least some of it goes in your body. And if it's not safe enough to swallow, why would you put it on your skin?

Allergic reactions create that immediate, visceral response that tells us something needs to stop. Hives might break out when a skin care product triggers the response, or something will burn or feel uncomfortable. But sometimes that response doesn't come right away. Sensitization can occur after prolonged use of a product with small amounts of an offending ingredient builds up until the skin rejects it. And sometimes, the damage is done without a single itch or bump.

Among the dozens of products we use on our skin—hand soap, body soap, shampoo, lotions, fragrances, cosmetics, treatments, not to mention the laundry soap and other secondary chemicals that make it to our skin from our clothes and homes—any one of them could be laced with several known toxicants. Triclosan, sulfates, phthalates, and parabens are among the most concerning. Fragrances can pose problems, as well. Unless you make your own products or purchase from a closely-trusted source, loose labeling requirements of many lesser-known harmful chemicals can leave potential concerns completely unknown.

Phthalates and parabens are known to disrupt the endocrine system, yet are still added to countless products on the shelves of our grocery stores and cosmetics cabinets. Researchers are digging for the extent of damage they can do—lotions and other products increase paraben and phthalate concentration in the urine of pregnant women, so what are the phthalates doing to the pregnancy and to the baby's future health? (Braun, et al, 2014) Adolescent girls who only used products free of these toxins saw urine concentrations drop significantly (by about half!) after just three days. (Harley, et al, 2016) What had the toxins already done to their development and health, and what happened if they returned to their former lotions and cosmetics after the study?

While researchers look for answers, the landscape of personal care products won't change unless consumers demand it. Manufacturers and makers can only develop what people want to buy, and until that looks like more natural, safer products, we'll only see more of the same. This is an instance where we can "vote with our dollars," supporting companies that refuse to include toxins that will sink into our skin and wash down our drains and into the water supply.

Household Products

Walk down the household aisle in the grocery store—you can smell exactly where you are. If you open the cabinets beneath your sink, you can probably smell the maelstrom of odor just as much. No one ever said the smell indicated something *healthy*, that's for sure. But at the same time, many of us don't think of these products as having an impact on health at all—right? Wrong.

We breathe the fumes, touch the surfaces, and live in environments soaked in toxic ingredients, many of which are hardly disclosed to consumers at all. The label might tell us all about the scent and the cleaning power, but little about the asthmatic and carcinogenic potential of their ingredients. (EWG, 2016) That pungent smell in the grocery store and under the cabinet is our warning: you don't want this stuff in your body!

If you are following the thread here, you'll notice a recurring theme: toxins aren't going to be banned, changed, or otherwise eliminated any time soon. There are new chemical compounds created and released all the time, with little labeling oversight and next to no official testing. Even what we unequivocally know to be dangerous is rarely banned. The onus is on the consumer to make their decisions based on labeling, trust in the maker of the product, and good use once it's in the home.

You might have already noticed the loud fragrances and cocktail of toxins in household cleaners lend to headaches and general malaise. They are not only harsh on "grime" as is so often projected, but they can be harsh on your body. The same problematic ingredients in personal care products are found in household cleaners, on top of bleach and harsh detergents.

Not all toxins come with labels, though, and our houses are full of them. We often hear that non-stick coatings on pans, for example, can leach PFCs into food if the coating is scratched, but we're exposed to the same chemicals in stain repellents, leather cleaners, even certain kinds of paper. (EPA, 2017) Furniture and other flame-retardant fabrics off-gas their chemicals into the air. Toys come coated in plastics and paints that can introduce your teething toddler to toxins like phthalates and lead. Even the insulation in the walls carries toxins that make their way into the air. Though the home itself is a concern we'll look at next, the products we bring into our homes can be much more easily controlled.

In the fascinating and eye-opening book *Slow Death by Rubber Duck: The Secret Danger of Everyday Things*, (Smith, 2011) the authors took this a step further and tested the effects of household products on themselves, wondering whether it was possible at all to avoid toxins. They did find that the levels of specifically targeted toxins—including BPAs, phthalates, pesticides, PFCs (non-stick coating), and others—could rise and fall quickly, much like the urinary phthalate levels in the adolescent girls we just talked about. (To really dive deep into the ways toxins can be controlled in a world where they can't be eliminated, *Slow Death by Rubber Duck* should be your next read.) Their conclusions suggest that we can make some change by choosing different products for cooking, cleaning, and furnishing.

However, they also had this to say in conclusion:

> *"Making different choices the next time you go to the grocery store can alleviate some of your family's pollution in the short term. But for a long-term fix, only improved government regulation and oversight of toxic chemicals is the answer. It's critical that we address this problem not only as consumers, but also as engaged citizens demanding better of their governments."*

In-Home Air Quality

For all of the things we can control, there's the looming knowledge that much more is out of our reach. This last source of toxins feels a lot like that. No matter what products we buy or eliminate, no matter what food we eat and water we drink, our homes are still the most toxic place to be. Hang in there, though—remember we aren't here to get overwhelmed and quit. Let's look at the reasons why.

We spend a lot of time indoors. We sleep with the windows shut, run heat and air units to regulate temperature (and circulate the same old air), wake to step outside just long enough for the morning commute and then get right back inside for school and work. Even errands take us from building to building. Within those buildings we have furniture and even electronics that off-gas their production chemicals. We have toxic cleaners and air fresheners. We have dust, which holds the remnants of all of those chemicals including phthalates and other endocrine-disruptors, blowing around and recirculating through our air vents. (Mitro, 2016) And as long as we keep our windows shut and we stay indoors, all of that flows through our lungs and distributes through our bodies.

And that's just the normal circumstances.

Extenuating circumstances lead to even more exposures. Any kind of moisture or water damage give way to mold growth. According to OSHA, "It is estimated that about 50 to 100 common indoor mold types have the potential for creating health problems." (OSHA, 2017) These exposures can be as irritating as runny nose and cough or as serious as contributing to the development of asthma in children.

Renovation, nearby construction, and new building projects bring air pollution all their own, filling the air with particles of dust, VOCs and other fumes, and countless chemicals in glues, plasters, paints, and more. But the most worrisome is that of lead dust. (WebMD, 2017) In older homes, layers of paint containing lead can be powdered into dust as walls are cut, sending lead particles flying through the air. This can be compounded by the constant risk of bringing lead dust into the home from old playgrounds and the dirt itself.

When indoor air quality is bad—and it is, more often than not—the consequences can be extensive. A home or workplace with poor air quality can lead to Multiple Chemical Sensitivity, which increases reactions to chemicals, or Sick Building Syndrome, which can look like a struggle with concentration, memory, and learning, as well as fatigue, nausea, headaches, asthma attacks, and overall malaise. (EPA, 2017)

Knowing that our homes aren't even a refuge from this chemical world, let's move onto some solutions that can help us mitigate the risks and create a better life now and in the future.

Solutions

We can't possibly state every source of toxins, list every toxicant, or give you a complete guide to a toxin-free life. It's just not possible. So we've focused on the major areas where singular, simple changes can make a big difference. For specific swaps for each category, read on to the Simple Swaps for Everyday Life guide found in the appendix.

Instead of being overwhelmed at the many sources of toxins in our lives, we hope your wheels are already turning, seeing areas where you can improve and become more efficient in the pursuit of whole-body, whole-life health for you and your family. To help you move in that direction, let's shift gears and talk specifically about the solutions you can start to implement today.

Minimize Exposure

The first and very best thing you can do is to minimize exposure. Wherever you've learned that toxins are a threat, look for a way to eliminate them or replace them with better choices. If you can put an in-home filter on your water source, you'll have made huge strides with that one move. A switch to home-made or safe, natural cleaning or personal care products will make a major difference, especially for your children. Changing eating habits will impact two of the 5 Essentials at once! If you can't buy organic, at least learn to wash your produce thoroughly and avoid the packaged food products. We have so little control over what is made, marketed, and distributed to the masses, but we can do our best within our own homes.

As for the question of our homes being toxic—don't get discouraged! There's plenty we can do there, too. **The first step is to simply get outside more.** Bring the outside air in with open windows and a break in air conditioning cycles. Spend some time taking walks, playing with your kids, and visiting with your neighbors for some fresh air. The next is to set up some nature-based air filtration by bringing plants indoors. Ivies and ferns, among dozens of other low-light plants, can effectively, measurably reduce the toxins in the air—including formaldehyde and mercury. (Claudio, 2011)

Perpetually Detox

Though we have a seemingly endless stream of new chemicals and toxicants to contend with today, history is quite familiar with toxins. One of the oldest forms of medicine—Ayurveda—hold detoxification as one of its core methods. In fact, Ayurvedic medicine even has a process for making sure their medicinal herbs are free of toxins themselves before they are used in the body. (Maurya, 2015) Traditional Chinese Medicine, another ancient practice, also had an understanding of detoxification, viewing it as a disturbance or interference usually removed with practices like acupuncture and acupressure. (Ceniceros, Brown, 1998)

As the years marched on, detoxification carried throughout religious, philosophical, and medical practices. There were ancient Biblical cleansing and dietary restrictions, bath-houses of Greece and Rome, saunas and sweat baths of Nordic and Native American traditions, and a recurring theme of removing exposure, encouraging natural detoxification processes, and utilizing botanical products.

After taking steps to minimize exposure, we have to turn inward to our own bodies and lifestyles to make sure the body has what it needs to process the rest. We rely on the body's innate ability to take care of itself. But we also know that the world and the modern lifestyle will overload those systems. Removing the obvious exposures that are within our control helps to balance the scales once again. Supporting the body's processes tips those scales even further in our favor.

Practicing the 5 Essentials will optimize your body's processes overall, which of course includes detoxification pathways. Chiropractic adjustments impact the nervous system, which controls all metabolic pathways, including detoxification pathways. Exercise moves the circulatory system more efficiently, helping the lungs expel air better and the blood to move freely as it carries both nutrients and toxins to the proper end-destinations.

In clinical practices, we often see clients struggling simultaneously with toxicity and weight loss. The two issues are frequently sides of the same coin. Losing fat gives the body less room to store excess toxins, and obesity tends to be connected with a toxic lifestyle. It should be noted that all those stored toxins will likely circulate the body while you are in the process of losing weight. (Merrill, et al, 2012) Be aware of this risk and what your body will need during the process. In the next chapter, we will dive deeper into supplementation as an added support in cases like these.

We can also add in steam and sauna rituals of the past, allowing the pores to open and expel whatever toxins they might harbor. Thoughtfulness pays off here, too—for instance, infrared saunas use non-toxic poplar wood, which is an important distinction when you hope to rid the body of toxins.

Eating a diet rich in antioxidants (all those colorful vegetables) can also help improve the body's natural process of scrubbing the cells and blood clean. Of all of the detox tricks out there, food is arguably the most powerful tool we have to support detoxification and remove this form of interference. (Hodges, Minich, 2015)

Good sleep, which we'll discuss with the mindset in chapter 8, is important not only for mental rest but to allow the body time to retreat away from constant, varying toxic exposures and eliminate all that the day has introduced. Careful, specific supplementation can also be used to support natural detoxification, which we will discuss more in the next chapter.

Clearly, the average North American has a sometimes overwhelming stack of toxic threats in their life. We also have many choices available to us to help mitigate those exposures. If you believe your toxin exposure extends beyond the average case, you will probably want to work with a care professional who is trained and experienced in detoxification. Your methods will look the same overall—removal of the threat, supporting the body, and adding botanical products—but may require more intensive steps to accomplish the same goals.

No matter your circumstances, choosing to do the next right thing for your household and your body will make a difference. Whether that looks like something as big as seeking help for advanced toxin exposure or something as small as washing your produce better, every little thing adds up to ease the burden of detoxification, allowing your body to finally, more thoroughly, minimize toxins.

I'm Removing Your Diagnosis Completely

Cynthia Nakeyar

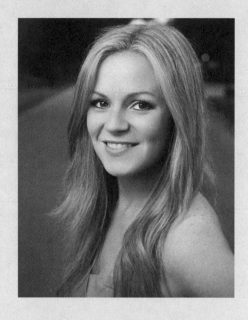

" In high school, I lacked motivation and frequently felt irritable with mood swings. I had been prescribed multiple psychotropic drugs for depression. At least once or twice a week, I got migraines so bad they sometimes affected my vision, and occasionally I had complete blackouts. My immune system and energy levels were low, I randomly napped throughout the day from sheer fatigue, and I caught a severe flu several times every year. I had severe stomach issues, and sometimes would have nausea and vomiting.

I also had severe lower back pain that woke me up at night. The pain was so bad, I couldn't vacuum or sleep for long periods without taking breaks.

Eventually, my doctor diagnosed me with ankylosing spondylitis—an arthritis affecting my lower back and pelvis.

My entire body felt stiff for an hour or longer when I woke up. My fingers were so swollen I often couldn't bend them. As a university student, this interfered with everything.

Altogether, I was miserable, and sick of being sick! I needed a big change.

Even though I had the diagnosis of ankylosing spondylitis, my doctors couldn't figure out why I had so much inflammation. At wit's end, I finally explored MaxLiving because my uncle had done so well on the program.

Having nothing to lose, I went all in with passion. I committed to following every one of the 5 Essentials. I got regular chiropractic adjustments. I strictly followed the Advanced Plan, eliminating all sugar, all grains, and even most fruits. I started burst training and weight training. I quit smoking and started taking nutrients. I went off birth control pills because I wanted my hormones to work naturally—I didn't want to interfere with them. I also jumped on the detox protocols with tons of veggies, plus charcoal and antioxidants along with my other supplements.

During this process, my family became closer. We all took the challenge to better our lives!

One year later, I've experienced a complete transformation in my health. I no longer need those random naps. I haven't had a headache in months. (I don't even remember the last one I had.) I no longer have blackouts. I haven't had a flu or cold this year, and I don't get nauseous.

Plus—my inflammation is gone! My rings are now oversized and don't fit me anymore. My shoe size has gone down, too.

I have very little lower back pain, and it doesn't wake me up at night anymore. In fact, I own a cleaning business now and am able to do lots of physical activity without pain. I can sit through long lectures and movies with no pain. My body doesn't feel stiff in the mornings these days.

As a nice "bonus," I've lost twenty pounds since starting the Advanced Plan. My concentration is much better, and my grades have improved by fifteen percent since last year. I'm more motivated and don't struggle with mood swings.

One of the best feelings was going to my doctor who had given me the diagnosis of ankylosing spondylitis three months after starting the program. She literally said, "I'm in shock!" and then she said, "I'm removing your diagnosis completely."

This is the best I've ever felt and the happiest I've ever been.

CHAPTER 7

Essential Supplementation

Before we get to the last of the 5 Essentials, we need to pause to discuss the matter of vitamins and supplements. A western philosophy of health looks for things that we can easily take—usually pills—that will make us feel better. Whether or not we actually *are* better is often irrelevant, as long as the noticeable symptoms are relieved. As we take steps toward a more complete sense of wellness, incorporating the 5 Essentials, sometimes the old philosophy stays with us. Vitamins and supplements seem to be the answer.

Unfortunately, too many "experts" and corporations are willing to take advantage of this tendency. And to great financial reward! In 2014, the Nutrition Business Journal reported more than $36 billion in estimated sales of vitamin and mineral supplements. (NIH, 2017) Nearly all of us can think back to how we might have contributed to that total, and for some of us, it was far too much. While it's wise to invest in quality supplements, it's unnecessary to spend hundreds of dollars each month on a countertop full of junk supplements and gimmicks.

Because we've been sold the lie that we need more supplements for more problems, the market has been flooded with all sorts of products and claims. New miracle cures and quick fixes are out on a regular basis, and old standbys—multivitamins and protein powders especially—are constantly reinvented into cheaper, tastier versions of themselves. Because this is a highly unregulated market, however, nearly anything can be packaged, labeled, and sold as a supplement.

There are dietary supplements that are absolutely worthwhile and will support your body as you work to remove interference and promote innate health. The most reliable way to find these supplements is to work with a nutritionist, dietary supplement specialist, or practitioner who can direct you to quality brands and exactly the products that you need. The more you can learn about supplements, the more you can engage in this aspect of wellness to make the best decisions for you and your family.

Supplements vs Varied Diets

After working through most of the 5 Essentials and making plans to implement them, you'll be passionate about the self-healing principles of chiropractic, nutrition, exercise, clean living, and—as we'll cover in the next chapter—mental focus. Knowing the potential that lies ahead when you've freed your body to be its absolute best, your steps forward will be motivated and effective. So when it comes to supplements, there are usually two directions people take: Some people decide that their diet provides all they need and choose not to supplement at all, while others carry their enthusiasm into their local nutrition store—or, worse, grocery store—and scoop up everything the representative—or, worse, someone online—tells them to buy.

As usual, the better path lies somewhere in the middle. Certainly, a good diet of varied, whole foods with plenty of vegetables and fruit is the first priority for getting the nutrients we need. But there are some practical gaps to fill (as well as some things we can't control) at play. Fully organic, relatively local food is not always available or affordable. In order to get the full benefits of food, a lot of factors have to be met that don't always line up for the average family. What's more, is that nutrient profiles aren't what they used to be. Back in 1999, the composition of dozens of foods were compared with records in 1950. (Davis, 1999) Protein, calcium, potassium, iron, vitamin C, and vitamin B12 were all lacking across the board. We've not improved our soil quality or farming standards since then—in fact, crops have been genetically modified to take more of a beating.

People who do use multivitamin supplements tend to have a better nutrient status than those who do not. On the other hand, they also report closer attention to nutrient intake overall than people who do not supplement. (Rock, 2007) There could be a chicken-and-egg situation here—which comes first, nutrition from dietary improvement or from the multivitamins? But healthy is healthy, and these are clearly tools that we can use to set our families on a trajectory of wellness.

What does this mean for the person or family in pursuit of MaxLiving? Sticking closely to your nutrition plans will take you a long way, but thanks to degrading food quality and the simple inhibitions of everyday life, you'll likely need some help getting the rest of the nutrients your body needs. This is the intended way to view vitamins, minerals, and other supplements—as things that *supplement* a healthy diet and lifestyle. Other reasons one might supplement might include a specific condition that needs extra attention to address, a specific dietary need that can't be met, or needing to meet the body halfway when a lifestyle concern like stress can't be avoided.

In other words, this is not a question of either/or, but of using both supplements and a varied diet in the most efficient way—in whatever way your body specifically needs.

Supplementing Nutrients

If someone tries to sell you a big bag of supplements, herbs, powders, and gimmicks, give each one a close look. "Sell" might be their priority more than supporting your health. There are some basic supplements that can be universally beneficial, however, and in those cases your due diligence will be to verify their quality, which we'll discuss more at the end of the chapter. These specific supplements provide nutrients that are easy to miss, or they support the body in repairing damage that's frequently done.

Multivitamin

The most common supplement and usually the first one we turn to is the a multivitamin which covers a wide range of nutrients in one bottle. Note that we aren't talking about one *pill*—more on that in a moment. For now, let's look at what multivitamins can do.

Though we need to have a balance of macronutrients—carefully-sourced fats, proteins, and carbs—vitamins and minerals are just as important as macronutrients. **Multivitamins are meant to bridge the micronutrient gap that busy lives and lacking food sources create.** Although there is no set definition for a multivitamin, and the industry comes with many regulatory gaps, it is broadly understood to be a supplement that contains a range of vitamins and minerals, without herbs or other substances. They are strictly intended to supplement a well-rounded diet to ensure inadequacies don't stack up.

Meeting this nutrient gap is important simply on manner of principle. Our bodies need the nutrition, and if it's within our power to provide it, we must! But there are some documented benefits to taking them, as well. In a thorough review published in 2014, researchers combed through multivitamin research for any effects on chronic illness. (Ward, 2014) With some caveats for existing nutrient status or other risk factors, they found a good deal of supportive evidence for multivitamins and the prevention or outcomes for anemia, eye health, and bone disease. There were even indications that cancer and heart disease prevention could be connected to multivitamins.

For compliance and easier study structures—among other reasons, no doubt—many of the existing multivitamin studies use a once-a-day supplement for their data. Optimal nutrient bases are more likely to be found in supplements that spread the contents out over several tablets or capsules. The trade off is a minor inconvenience when taking the supplement in exchange for better bioavailability and a higher quality composition. Beware any multivitamin that claims to provide a day's worth of nutrients in a single pill, gummy, sip, or treat.

Greens

Hang with me here. Greens supplements used to taste awful, even within the last decade. But it's worth giving them another chance. Most greens are great now. If you find one that you don't love, find another formulation. In fact, they are so good that if you are used to drinking sodas, coffee, and tea, they can flavor your water. Go for a bit of low-to-no-calorie greens instead of those artificially-sweetened flavor packets.

Dark, leafy green vegetables are powerhouses of nutrition. Nearly a multivitamin in their own right, they contain carotenoids, vitamins C and K, folate, iron and calcium, as well as a good amount of fiber. (Adams, 2013) They are also excellent sources of iron and antioxidants. If you could add one salad filled with dark, leafy greens every day, you'd be healthier already—but do you actually do that? Would your kids? **Greens are often lacking in Western diets.** If this is true for you, a greens powder is probably a beneficial, if not required, supplement.

If you drink smoothies, protein shakes, or homemade meal replacements at all, make sure you can add greens to them. That way, you can increase the vegetable content without losing flavor or complicating the recipe.

Usually powered but sometimes extracted, greens supplements are just that: greens. Children, people with sensory issues, and those who are new to eating well and are learning to enjoy things like greens can all benefit from this benign way to boost your nutrient profile. Add the liquid or powder to smoothies and shakes, water, or sprinkle it into soups and other dishes. The healthier you become after the addition of greens and a focus on the 5 Essentials, the easier it will be to add in salads and other sources of greens. The great thing about greens, though, is that you can't really have too many.

Vitamin D3

Unlike the nutrients we've discussed so far, vitamin D doesn't actually come from food. Our bodies produce it when exposed to the sun's rays. So the same lifestyle that keeps us inside toxic buildings all day long, sitting at desks or sitting at home, can also alter our nutrient status. For this reason—as well as genetic make-up, since melanin can block access to vitamin D even when you're outside—vitamin D status can vary from person to person. Your practitioner can test you to let you know what your levels are so that you know how you might need to supplement.

Without adequate vitamin D, calcium and phosphorous can't be absorbed well. Bones might begin to weaken—the classic deficiency shows up as rickets, characterized by a bowing shapes to bones, especially in the legs. Muscles can begin to weaken, which can lead to more falls on those weakened bones. These effects demonstrate its function on bone health and muscular development, though its day to day use reaches even further. Vitamin D mirrors a steroid hormone, affecting not only the structural systems of the body but also the gut, cardiovascular system, brain, and immune system. We're still learning how this plays out in specific diseases, but with each of those functions supported, you can imagine the possibilities. Depression and cognitive function, autoimmune disorders, protection against communicative diseases, and eye health have all been connected to low levels of vitamin D. Yet we still find people from childhood to adults at high risk for vitamin D deficiency. (Nair, 2012)

Vitamin D3 in particular—the form it takes once the body has converted the sunlight—is the supplement of choice, giving your body exactly what it needs without the middleman of absorption and breakdown or conversion. One professor's essay published in 2010 summarizes the dire situation we're in without vitamin D3:

"Vitamin D3 deficiency can result in obesity, diabetes, hypertension, depression, fibromyalgia, chronic fatigue syndrome, osteoporosis and neuro-degenerative diseases including Alzheimer's disease. Vitamin D deficiency may even contribute to the development of cancers, especially breast, prostate, and colon cancers. Current research indicates vitamin D deficiency plays a role in causing seventeen varieties of different cancers as well as heart disease, stroke, autoimmune diseases, birth defects, and periodontal disease. Vitamin D3 is believed to play a role in controlling the immune system (possibly reducing one's risk of cancers and autoimmune diseases), increasing neuromuscular function and improving mood, protecting the brain against toxic chemicals, and potentially reducing pain." (Naeem, 2010)

Very few foods can stand in for sunlight. Egg yolks and beef liver make the very short list, which of course should both be sourced from sustainable farms that feed their animals well. Because of the urgency that vitamin D deficiency creates and because we cannot measure our intake including the variables that help or hinder conversion of sunlight to vitamin D, supplementation is often necessary.

There is a point where vitamin D—measured with a serum test called 25-hydroxyvitamin D—becomes too high, but this can only happen with over-supplementation. Most of us are at or below optimal ranges for vitamin D. There is only a range and various stances on what true the true optimal amount is, not a hard and fast rule.

Even so, the current RDA is only 800 IUs. (NIH, 2017) Researchers in Switzerland have found that the general population can take anywhere from 1,400-4000 IUs without adverse effects. (Bischoff-Ferrari, 2009) Natural health advocates typically reach for more like 5,000-10,000 IUs, and have a slightly higher goal for serum levels. If you're concerned about deficiency, check with your practitioner to determine your vitamin D status, then supplement with vitamin D3 to feed your body what it needs to combat the correlated risks.

Probiotics

Bacteria are not simply germs or enemies, but a complex world of microorganisms that function alongside us every day. They are in and on our bodies, covering every surface, part of every environment. **We hold a symbiotic relationship with**

bacteria. In a healthy body, they partner with the immune system, digestive system, and even the skin to drive us toward health.

Everything we eat affects the bacteria levels in the gut and throughout the body, either partnering with bacteria or working against them. The gut, then, becomes a center of bacterial activity in the body, which is not a coincidence given that the gut is also a center of immune response. (Fields, 2015)

Probiotic foods are fermented, and there are many ways to add that to your diet. Usually, we think of kombucha, yogurt, or yogurt-based drinks, but fermentation opens almost endless doors for vegetables and vegetable dishes such as kimchi, homemade sauerkraut, and almost any type of lacto-fermented pickled vegetable. We're looking for tons of bacteria in all sorts of varieties, not a single serving of sugared-up yogurt. If your diet doesn't have lots of cultured foods—the kinds of foods people have thrived on for centuries—you probably could use a daily probiotic supplement.

As a supplement, probiotics are usually a liquid, sometimes powdered-and-encapsulated concoction of bacteria cultures that are taken on an empty stomach. Because they are live cultures, a good probiotic would need to be refrigerated. They should also contain billions—yes, *billions*—of active cultures and a wide variety of bacterial strains.

Both gut-friendly foods and probiotic supplements are recommended for anyone, and there are many health conditions that probiotics help the body to combat. Whenever the gut and the immune system are involved, probiotics should be considered. Researchers in Pakistan reviewed the body of literature on probiotics to identify the most effective uses. (Singh, 2013) They're indicated for diarrhea of many causes, IBS and IBD, allergies, UTI—even oral health like bad breath and gum and teeth health could benefit from certain applications of probiotics.

Bacteria are here to stay, and it's necessary for our bacteria population to be ruled by the beneficial strains. Feeding the body high quality, gut-friendly foods, avoiding high sugar content that might feed detrimental bacteria, and avoiding antibiotics except when absolutely necessary are all important components of a gut-friendly life. Probiotics are the next step, and one that just about everyone could stand to take.

Omega-3

We've talked about eating lots of *good* fats, but what does it mean for a fat to be good? Essential fatty acids (EFAs) are categorized by their molecular structure, with omega 3 and omega 6 taking center stage. The word *essential* here only means that the body cannot produce it. For example, there are omega 9 fatty acids, but those are not essential because the body can synthesize them in other ways.

The body does need both types of EFAs. Either type can be damaged or not, but omega 6 types, even in their undamaged states, have become so prevalent in our diets full of meats and processed foods that there is absolutely no reason to try to consume it intentionally. In fact, as we discussed in the chapter on nutrition, the optimal ratio of omega 6 to omega 3 is dramatically lower than what we actually consume. (Bartnikowska, et al, 1997) In these quantities, omega 6 EFAs begin to be harmful, producing inflammation in the body.

A stabilization of the ratio between these types of EFAs can help free the body to address many conditions. While the nutrition aspect of the 5 Essentials moves us toward a lower omega 6 consumption, it's still unlikely that diet alone can foster the balance. There are simply too many of one with not enough of the other in our daily lives. Supplementation—bridging the nutritional gaps beyond the efforts you're already making—to increase omega 3 consumption becomes vital.

Choosing the right omega 3 supplement is important, particularly when you recall that toxins are stored in fat. Fish provide one of the most prolific sources of omega 3 fatty acids, but fish are often farmed and bred and even caught in mercury-contaminated waters. Once the supplement is extracted, it needs to be protected from rancidification, which can go unnoticed in a gel capsule or to the untrained consumer. (Cameron-Smith, et al, 2015) A good omega 3 supplement will extract its sources—often a combination of plant and animal sources for diversification—through a carefully filtered, carefully protected process.

When the imbalance of EFAs is corrected, the body can begin to address a range of problems. Mental health is a prominent concern, given that the brain is so heavily fueled by fats. A growing body of evidence is sorting out how best to use omega 3s for things like depression and cognitive function, with promising results. Most often, it's women who see the most relief from depression symptoms when they add an omega 3 supplement, though there are many studies that suggest its use with dementia, stress-related depression, and other mental health concerns. (Wani, et al, 2015) The anti-inflammatory nature of omega 3s plus a restored ratio also lends itself to cardiovascular protection and a slowed inflammatory response—for pregnant women, the effect extends to the unborn baby and their future health, as well. (Swanson, et al, 2012)

Because it's so specific to an individual, the only way to know your personal balance of omega fatty acids would be to have your levels tested. As a general rule, though, your diet can give you a pretty reliable clue. If you're loaded down with grains, processed foods, or even soy and corn—you probably have more than enough omega 6. The cleaner your diet, the more likely an omega 6 addition to your supplement regimen could be helpful.

Detox Supplements

The next of the 5 Essentials that is often supplemented with natural products is that of detoxification. Once we decide to eliminate toxic inputs in our lives and free our cells and processes of the effects of toxins, all of the voices selling detox products become amplified. If we weren't before, we suddenly become aware of all of the teas, plans, pills, and juices on the market that claim to strip your body of toxins.

Tread with caution.

Fads and trends are often ill-conceived, and can actually create even more of a problem when they deprive us of the nutrients we need to support healthy, natural detoxification. Your liver and kidneys, as well as immune and excretory systems (including sweat!) are constantly working to keep you clear of toxins. **Our job is to support the body's detoxification systems rather than subvert, replace, or force them.**

Antioxidants

On a cellular level—not just filtered out of blood or excreted through sweat, but gathering and dealing with toxins within each cell—antioxidants are the key to detoxification. The toxic components of our environments are called *free radicals*, and antioxidants are their Kryptonite. Free radicals create oxidative stress, which we know to be associated with disease and damage to the body. Antioxidants are so named because they mitigate that damage.

The best way to increase antioxidant intake is through a diet full of rich, colorful vegetables and fruits. You can't eat too many of these foods, which means there's no limit to the cell-scrubbing power you can pack into salads and snacks. On the other hand, selective, high-dose supplementation of specific antioxidants like beta carotene and vitamin E have been linked with worse, even deadly outcomes. (NIH, 2016) So, the first place to go for antioxidants is the diet itself. When you need to supplement, you can work with an herbalist or trained nutritionist or supplement specialist who can help guide your intake.

One antioxidant supplement that could be useful without the risk of fat soluble vitamin intake is glutathione. An intra-cellular antioxidant, glutathione works within the cell out, rather than influencing or forcing actions from the external. Within the cell, glutathione attaches to the carcinogens, heavy metals, herbicides, pesticides, and more, and then converts it into water-soluble material that can be excreted.

Although—or because—glutathione is one of the best substances the body can use to eliminate heavy metals like mercury, those exposures and eliminations deplete glutathione stores. (Patrick, 2002) The more glutathione we use, the less we have available, and depletion can lead to neurological damage, not to mention a loss of a major source of antioxidant action.

Years ago, different food types were measured for their glutathione content. Uncooked fruits and vegetables ranked highest, cooked produce lost some; and dairy, grains, and processed foods contained very little. (Wierzbicka, 1989) So again, dietary focus can be helpful. But is it enough? Some specific foods might not contain glutathione directly, but can metabolize into it. Sulphur-containing cruciferous vegetables like broccoli and cauliflower make the list—noted in an evaluation that lists them as lowering the risks for certain cancers. (Joseph, 2004)

Glutathione can be restored by supplementation, a point that researchers recently evaluated over a six-month trial. (Richie, et al, 2014) In addition to the restored glutathione, markers of the immune system increased alongside direct glutathione supplementation. The glutathione numbers began to drop again after a month of discontinued use, however, so supplementation should be considered for long-term use or while dealing with an exposure that would otherwise deplete your stores.

There are several ways to accomplish glutathione supplementation, and the best option might be different from person to person. N-Acetyl Cysteine (NAC) is a relatively common supplement and a precursor to glutathione. It does not appear to create a long term increase, however, and can require high doses (400-1200 mg/day). Direct glutathione can be supplemented as an intra-oral spray, bypassing much of the digestive tract, or in modified compounds. Liposomal glutathione combines it with liposomes to ensure it survives digestion and reaches the cells. Acetylated glutathione also survives the gut, then goes a step further by including cellular enzymes to further ensure absorption with minimal effort from the body. Both of these are dosed lower than NAC, and are highly absorbable. Your practitioner can evaluate your needs to identify the best option for your body.

The only universal action we can take to improve glutathione—and all detoxification systems, really—is to exercise regularly. When researchers evaluated eighty sedentary people without obvious disease, aerobic and circuit training together improved the glutathione antioxidant process and stores in the body. (Elokda and Nielson, 2007) It's another instance where we see the 5 Essentials working with one another to accomplish similar purposes, and supplementation is an option only when necessary.

Elemental Detox

Heavy metals are borne of the earth, so it seems right that we draw from the earth to address them. Substances that would naturally interact with each other in the ground might have similar effects in the body. Ayurvedic medicine relies on clays for detoxification, as have countless traditions throughout the centuries.

As always, however, safety and efficacy are our first priorities. As detox products have shifted into the limelight of trends and marketing buzzwords, clays and powders are sold to us as near magic. **It's important to always know what you are supplementing with and why, and that's even truer with clays and powders.** This is a step beyond consuming healing foods or encapsulated nutrients and should be taken with a full understanding of the process.

There are a few fascinating substances that directly support the body's detoxification process. Activated charcoal, bentonite clay, and diatomaceous earth are part of the detox toolbox that the earth harbors for us.

Medically, activated charcoal is used in an emergency case of acute poisoning or toxicity, meant to draw the toxin out and expel it. (NIH, 2017) The written record of charcoal to absorb and draw out poisons reaches back to the 1700s and early 1800s. Its unique ability to thoroughly draw toxins out of the body and into itself without harming the GI tract makes it invaluable for any toxin that moves through the gut. (Derlet and Albertson, 1986)

External, regular use on the skin can help draw toxins out and assist in the skin's barrier functions. Toothpaste and dental preparations using activated charcoal can also be used regularly. Internally, a periodic cleansing or detoxification support routine can benefit from the addition of charcoal pills. In lower doses than a medical-grade intervention, the tablets are meant to make a clean sweep through the body, removing whatever they can gain access to. Because of the potency of activated charcoal, however, make sure to only take this an hour or two apart from meals, vitamins, or medications so that the charcoal doesn't have any nutrients or drugs to bind to.

Modern use of bentonite clay draws from centuries of traditional uses of clay as a skin, hair, and internal cleanser. A 2017 review evaluated the results of the body of scientific studies done on bentonite clay, compiling the benefits and uses that we might draw from. (Moosavi, 2017) It noted gastrointestinal health without altering mineral absorption or gut flora, skin health in masks and topical treatments, as well as the ability to absorb and mitigate toxins. The caution with internal use of clay is that it can absorb electrolytes, which could be detrimental in high doses. If you're taking bentonite clay for the purpose of detoxification, it should be under the guidance and supervision of a qualified practitioner.

Diatomaceous earth is the powdered remains of aquatic fossils. It is an excellent purifier—scrubbing water clean when added to filters, acting as an antiparasitic for chickens, and functioning as an insecticide or pesticide used sparingly in organic gardens and for home use. (Farrah, 1991) (Bennett, et al, 2011) (Hosseini, et al, 2014)

Still, diatomaceous earth is more or less just silica. You might recall silica as a workplace toxin that can leave workers with chronic lung disease. (Rushton, 2007) That's because diatomaceous earth can be made into crystalline compounds— usually for commercial use—or amorphous compounds, which are usually food-grade or GRAS (generally recognized as safe). The crystalline version is by far the most concerning, and when it becomes airborne and ingested into the lungs, the sharp edges of the tiny material scrape and scratch the lungs, leading to lung disease, even connected with cancer. (UCONN, 2017) As for amorphous, GRAS silica, the data is extremely limited and largely seems to indicate safety, but the limitations keep us from knowing the exact risks. (Merget, 2002) We do know that silica itself is a nutrient that the body needs, so at the very minimum, diatomaceous earth should be used with caution when viewed as a source of those nutrients. Only food grade powder should be used, and only in small amounts mixed into water. Never dry, to prevent the risk of aspiration, and don't "puff" it into the air or lean over the container to breathe it.

This said: detox supplements meant to enhance or assist the body's natural processes should not be taken lightly or without a thorough understanding of their proper uses and inherent risks.

Finally, though not an element but nonetheless powerful: milk thistle provides a simple, daily support of the liver—our most important detox organ. If clays and charcoal are meant to assist the body by removing threats, milk thistle is meant to recruit reinforcements for the attack. The liver has a lot of work to do as it cleanses the blood. Fatty acids, alcohol, sugars, and toxins only add to the load, slowing the process and risking long term health. Look for a milk thistle supplement with an 80% standardized silymarin content—the active ingredient that will support your body through the daily detox routine as well as in case of more dire detox needs.

Supplementing Exercise

The fitness industry has co-opted supplements in many ways, with millions of dollars in pills, powders, and drinks sold to people in the name of performance. Because supplements lack quality control regulations, a manufacturer can promise a great deal more than they are required to deliver, leaving consumers with a countertop covered in pre-, mid , and post workout products that can be unnecessary at best and dangerous at worst.

Protein supplements are the biggest culprit, used as meal replacements and workout enhancers alike. Though there are health benefits to protein—whey in particular—the big business side of it has diluted quality to a point of major concern. Not only are the commercial whey powders sourced in conventional (read: questionable) farming circumstances, but then they are processed and modified into oblivion on order to fill those massive megastore tubs. Other red flags that your protein is bad are high contents of sugar or—more often and arguably worse—artificial sweeteners, corn derivatives, dyes, and artificial flavors. You also have to watch for high-heat processed whey, which can create a denatured, unstable product once in the body. (Jeewanthi, 2015)

Protein supplements do have their place. A whey protein diet has long been acknowledged for its glutathione support, and it really can help the body to recover from exercise. (Bounous, et al, 1989) (Brown, et al, 2017) A realistic view of what protein supplements can and cannot do, as well as the quality of the product you choose, can help you to use these supplements to effectively support exercise as part of the 5 Essentials.

Pure Protein is Never a Meal

Think about the last meal that you ate. What types of food were on your plate? Good or bad isn't even the question here, so much as composition. You probably had a decent selection of food groups. Let's ignore most of them. Look only at the protein you ate. Was it completely lean, or were there traces of fat? How about minerals? We could go as far as to wager that not one person reading this book had a completely pure protein on their dinner plates, unless they had replaced a meal with a protein supplement.

The next question we have to ask ourselves then, is *why*? Why don't our proteins come completely separate from other nutrients? Better yet, let's reframe it: If our foods are integrated with a range of nutrients, how can we replace an entire range of nutrients with one, single, extracted, pure component and still call it a meal?

On principle, restricting nutrients runs counter to the MaxLiving goals we've outlined. If we trust our bodies to thrive when free of interference, we have to provide them an environment to thrive within. This includes eating a range of nutrient-dense foods throughout the day. Even if intermittent fasting and a smaller window for mealtime works best for you, you should still consume the nutrients your body would have needed throughout the whole day, only in a smaller window. Nutrient restriction doesn't remove interference at all.

Instead, whey protein and pure proteins should be *supplementing* your normal path toward the 5 Essentials. It can be used to boost intake when you need to gain weight or support recovery when working to lose it. Scientific literature tells us protein supplements are connected with both weight loss and better cardiovascular health. (Wirunsawanya, 2017) So go ahead and use protein to bolster the nutrient content of a smoothie. But it cannot replace the complex carbs, good fats, and caloric content that a full meal provides.

Plant vs. Animal Protein

When you think of protein, what type of food do you envision? Most people jump straight to animal protein, and sometimes think that's all there is. Case in point: vegans are often chastised for not having a protein source. In reality, a diet rich in varied vegetables can sufficiently—though perhaps not easily, depending on your familiar eating habits—provide your body with the protein that you need. The same is true for protein supplements: whey is *not* your only option!

Researchers in France took this concept to task when they evaluated whey protein and pea protein against each other and a placebo. (Babault, 2015) For twelve weeks, all of the participants (more than 150 men) underwent a physical training regimen. Some took pea protein powder, some took whey, and some were given a placebo. By the end of the trial, both protein groups had increased muscle thickness and strength compared to placebo.

Whey is a naturally-separated liquid that drains off as a byproduct of cheese production. Once it gained attention as a health product instead of a waste product, the commercial wheels were set in motion. First, powdered and filtered whey concentrate allowed for it to be more shelf-stable for storage and shipping. After that, consumers expected a consistent product in texture, flavor, and protein alone. Isolate became the answer, but at the expense of other nutrients. If you choose to use whey protein, concentrate provides more well-rounded nutrient objectives, and an organic, carefully sourced product is vital. Make sure the grassfed cows aren't fed grass that's been sprayed with pesticides!

Or, you can simply switch to a plant-based protein powder like pea protein to gain the same benefits without the drawbacks and sourcing issues. Plant protein absorbs slower, as well, so when you do add it to a smoothie for a quick, portable, easy-nutrition meal, you'll get a better return than whey.

Other Supplements to Consider

We've covered some of the supplements that just about everyone can benefit from, and outside of that, many of the gimmicks and heavily marketed products are simply unnecessary. But every person is different, and there will likely be some other supplements you come across that can be conditionally beneficial. The best way to know whether you need a supplement is to work with a nutritionist or other qualified practitioner who can assess your needs and match you with the best solution.

Magnesium

Have you ever wondered at the amount of nutrition they can pack into multi-supplements? All of the vitamins and minerals, sometimes with herbs as well, into a few pills. It is a wonder, but physics are still a factor. Magnesium is a bulky mineral, so even the best supplements will not often contain optimal amounts. Meanwhile, magnesium deficiency is under-diagnosed, prevalent, and—as noted in 2010—associated with eleven of the major health conditions our society struggles against. (Ismail, 2010)

Without sufficient magnesium, neurological functions cannot be performed, heart tones and rhythm will be weak, bones will be weak, and muscles will not contract and relax well. Magnesium regulates cell energy, electrolyte balance, and contributes to glutathione production. As vital as it is, magnesium sources are poor in the developed world. Processed foods and demineralized water have replaced many of our sources of magnesium. Spring or mineral water, green vegetables, legumes, meat, and fish will increase magnesium intake, but sometimes supplementation is helpful or necessary in order to replenish nutrient stores. (Jahnen-Dechent and Ketteler, 2012)

Magnesium supplements are most commonly found in pill, liquid, or powder form. The more readily absorbable your supplement is, the better the body will be able to use it. When the magnesium is coupled with an amino acid—"chelated" magnesium, as in the case of magnesium glycinate, malate, and taurate—it can be accessed more readily. Your practitioner can help you to identify the exact type of magnesium that is best for your needs.

Adrenal support

Herbs border on the line between food and medicine, and there are many potential herbal supplements for a range of health concerns. Without verging into an allopathic treatment philosophy, there are some supportive herbs that you may find helpful. Milk thistle, for example, is an herb that we've mentioned already as detox support. As a liver-supportive herb, milk thistle can be protective or restorative, allowing the liver to return to normal function.

An entire class of herbs that should be on your radar is that of *adaptogens*. Named for their ability to normalize the body, helping it to adapt to stress and other circumstances as seamlessly as possible, adaptogens are immensely helpful for today's lifestyles. Astragalus is an adaptogen you might have heard of already, because it's often paired with Echinacea as an immune-regulator. Ashwagandha is another important adaptogen, which has been used for centuries in Ayurvedic medicine. Ashwagandha is neuroprotective, anti-inflammatory, and helps with stress adaptation, among many other effects. Specifically, tests have indicated it can affect cortisol levels directly, slowing the stress response and supporting the adrenals. (Singh, et al, 2011)

There are many adaptogens and other herbs available to support the body and mind through times of stress. Again, the key is to work with someone who is fluent in herbalism and familiar with your circumstances in order to direct you to the best choices.

CoQ10

Another strong antioxidant, coenzyme Q10 is most often used to specifically support heart health. In the diet, CoQ10 is found in foods that few people consume regularly—organ meat, oily fish—as well as whole grains, which pose problems of their own when it comes to sourcing, preparation, and nutrient availability. In other words, most of this region is eating low-quality bread and passing on the liver and onions, so it's not unreasonable to assume we're missing out on CoQ10, too.

Although researchers haven't found universal benefits for everyone to take this supplement, there are some demographics that are especially susceptible to loss of the enzyme. (Saini, 2011) Athletes, for example, need all of their cells to consume and use oxygen efficiently. CoQ10 works right in the mitochondria—the energy production portion of the cell—and performance will falter if stores are low. The elderly also tend toward deficiency, as well as people taking statins for cholesterol.

B-Complex

Nutrition as we know it looks very different from what was known only a few generations ago. The discovery of macronutrients came first, acknowledging that the body needs a balance of protein, fat, and carbs to thrive. Then micronutrients came in the 19th and 20th centuries, as microscopes and other developments allowed scientists to break things down into components. **Vitamins were so named because they were vital to life, and as they were discovered, they were named.** However, the alphabetical naming convention started after a "vitamin B" was named for its ability to cure Beri Beri. Vitamin A came next, then C and D, then E. The trend continued, but molecules were denoted as vitamins then later determined not to be.

As the discovery and refining knowledge of vitamins grew, B vitamins were first grouped together and numbered because they performed similar actions. Each was a water soluble coenzyme. As more about their structure and actions was discovered, the B vitamins were given their own names apart from the numbered conventions, and those names are used more and more today. You're more likely to hear "riboflavin" than B2, though B6 and B12 are more commonly used than pyridoxine and cobalamin, respectively.

Vitamins in the B complex family are often antioxidant, neuroprotective, and mood stabilizing. Because our cells interact with nutrients at receptor sites, supplementing with one without balancing the others can lead to deficiencies in other areas, so a B complex is preferred over individual supplementation. For added bioavailability, methylated versions are excellent choices. Methylfolate bypasses the body's process for breaking the nutrient down into usable form, which is helpful for anyone and could be vital for people whose bodies cannot perform that function on their own. B12 is frequently given as a shot, though high doses orally can be just as effective. (Butler, 2006) B vitamins should also be methylated, for the same reason.

Up to a third of the population has the genetic variant known as MTHFR, which— among other things—prevents the body from turning some of the B-complex vitamins into a usable form. This can lead to symptoms ranging from unpleasant to life-altering. You can ask for a test to determine whether you have this genetic variant, but a good first step is to choose bioavailable, methylated sources of B-complex and folate no matter what. (MAYO, 2017)

B vitamins as a group can be found in a variety of foods, but B12 in particular is primarily sourced in animal products, leaving vegans highly vulnerable to deficiency.(Langan, 2017) B12 can also become low if intestinal issues like gastric acid or irritable bowel disease inhibit nutrient absorption, if you take medications like metformin that are known to deplete stores, or in old age. The serum numbers in a blood draw are not always accurate, so watch for fatigue, depression or anxiety, general pain and discomfort, weakness or dizziness, digestive problems, and focus or cognitive problems.

Quality is Paramount

For all of the benefits to be gained, nothing that we've talked about in this chapter matters if supplements aren't carefully chosen for quality. The basic standards that manufacturers are meant to adhere to have little to do with the actual content of the supplement. We already know that nutrient levels vary under a range of circumstances from growth to processing, and the same is true for supplement preparation.

Make sure your supplement manufacturer produces pharmaceutical grade products, standardized where possible, with transparency in their quality testing. Milk thistle, for example, is most effective when standardized to 80% silymarin content. A manufacturer testing that content will have a tighter rein on the actual product than one that does not.

Supplements are much closer to the growth process than actual pharmaceuticals, and it's important for the products to be grown organically. This, again, has an impact on the composition of the supplement, as well as safety. Other safety concerns include proper dosing. Fat-soluble vitamins will be stored in the body when taken in excess rather than eliminated with other water content. That storage can become dangerously toxic.

On the other hand, dosing sizes can be pitifully low, as well. A manufacturer intending to capitalize on the market has little invested in the actual results of the product and much invested in you feeling comfortable taking lots of pills and buying more bottles. Be familiar with the type of supplement you need, how much your body needs, and the best way you will be able to absorb it. The label on the back will not likely get all of those things right, which leads to the final note about vitamins, minerals, supplements, and herbs:

When in doubt, find a professional. Not the first person who appears in the grocery store aisle, but someone who can sit down with you and your health history to help you fill the gaps that the 5 Essentials have left. Shifting toward each of these Essentials is a big step for most of us, and it's bound to be difficult on the mind and body. When used properly and effectively, supplements are useful tools to support you on the journey toward true MaxLiving.

Trading My Cane for Racing Gear
Peggy Motil

" For over a decade, I suffered. My muscles and joints hurt non stop. I would have headaches that would last a month at a time. The swelling and pain in my legs caused me to limp all week at work. Mentally, I lived in a fog. I struggled to make decisions and, sometimes, just to find words. I experienced constipation daily.

Trying to figure out what was wrong with me, I was having blood work done every six months—I felt like a human pin cushion. I had numerous brain scans. Plenty of doctors told me that "it was all in my head." Along with way, I was diagnosed with restless legs syndrome and Hashimoto's disease, but I knew there was more going on.

As part of the Hashimoto's diagnosis, my primary doctor explained that I would need to take Synthroid for the rest of my life. My body was seeing my thyroid as an enemy and would attack it until it was gone. True autoimmunity. I tried the nutrition route and the supplement route, but nothing improved.

I began having anxiety attacks. I was simply losing hope. I was then diagnosed with fibromyalgia and my gallbladder started dysfunctioning. Testing showed that my gallbladder was only functioning at 34% and needed to be removed. I started to question if God had forgotten me. I had to begin using a cane to get around.

My family suffered watching me live in pain.

I had a mission trip scheduled to Haiti, but through a mix of circumstances, the trip was canceled. Serendipitously, I was invited on a mission trip the same week to the Dream Center in Los Angeles—and I went. My travel partner, Summer, was practicing the 5 Essentials under the guidance of her chiropractor, and because MaxLiving had just opened a clinic in the Dream Center, she sought out its care while we were there for the mission trip. For days, Summer urged me to get myself checked. I resisted. I told summer that there was no way my fibromyalgia could have anything to do with my spine. But Summer was relentless—and I went in for an examination.

The chiropractor looked at me, ran some tests and said, "I bet you feel like you have little bombs going off in your body." I began to cry because that is exactly how I had described it to others. I received my first adjustment. This brought immediate relief to my digestive system.

After the mission trip, I sought out a chiropractor for follow-up care in my hometown. I had structural X-rays taken. Causes of my problems were starting to become understood. I started with care. After my second or third adjustment, the pain in my shoulders that had been there for two to three years vanished. I realized there was something to this!

I was very faithful to my appointments and to doing all of my home exercises. The team helped me with my nutrition and I started the Advanced Plan right away. For three months, I followed the plan religiously, plus I did juice and liver cleanses, and started a new regimen of supplements. I began losing weight and feeling better. My thyroid started to function normally—my diagnosis was removed and I was able to come off the medication for it.

I went from collecting canes to completing a three-mile Terrain Race with twenty-four obstacles! My life was restored.

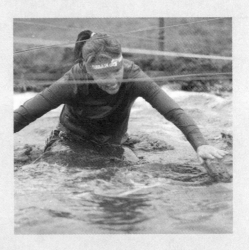

My daughter started, too; she no longer has migraines and her immune system is strong for the first time.

My husband started, and he no longer takes blood pressure medication. He's lost thirty-five pounds.

My brother started; he was already healthy and wants to stay that way.

...and I'm now the office manager for the clinic that changed my life.

CHAPTER 8
Mindset for Life

Although there are certain aspects of the 5 Essentials that might be easier to address than others—starting to visit a chiropractor regularly requires little effort for great return, for example—there isn't really a hierarchy within them. It is difficult to say that one essential is more important than the other. After all, they are each *essentials*. So as the last that we'll cover in this book, mindset is certainly not the least important. In fact, for many of us, it will need to be a focus long before we've eliminated toxins, changed our eating habits, or anything else.

Sometimes, the condition of the mind keeps us from taking any steps forward at all. Conversely, it is often a change in mindset that propels you to read a new book (like this one), make nutritional changes, commit to a fitness plan, or anything else to transform health over time.

But, to establish the state of your mind right now, check in with yourself. As you've read through this book, how have you reacted to the goals and suggestions we've put forth? Did you read about interval training and think, "I'm not the kind of person who *trains*." Were you excited about a more nutrient-dense diet, or did you think of all the foods you could never give up? How many times did you think you could *never* or would *always* do a certain thing? For all of the times you've started a new routine and then stopped, what have you told yourself?

Each time we utter a definitive statement—*always, never, can't, won't*—we limit ourselves. These limiting beliefs restrict our potential. Look around at how many people in your life are stressed, tired, depressed, and down on themselves. We're burned out, worn out, and giving out.

A MaxLiving life flows from a mindset of wellness. There are practical ways to adapt our bodies to a mindset of wellness, and there are tangible consequences when we don't. Similarly, there are more abstract ways to change our outlook on life, affecting both the practical and the spiritual. The lofty "I think, therefore I am," and the pithy "you are what you eat" fall on level ground with this essential. Wherever we set our minds, whatever we believe to be true and dwell on as reality, begins to shape our lives—for better or worse.

The Stressed Out Mind

I'm so stressed.

Just a little stressed right now.

Stressing over this right now!

We throw the word *stress* around so casually. It's become an expected part of life—one that we just deal with until we finally get to take vacation or maybe when we retire. So, onward we go, pushing through the exhaustion as long as we can. But the crash comes no matter how much we want to keep going. If not by an acute illness, then slowly by chronic disease—stress will wear us down until we are ill.

Biologically speaking, stress is anything that affects homeostasis. Whatever shifts the body off balance is a stress. This of course includes the things we normally consider to be stress—workplace pressure, finances, busy schedules that keep us working and worries—as well as some things we'd consider to be healthy. Heavy training and endurance exercise are stress, too, as far as the body is concerned. Stress, by this definition, triggers failsafe mechanisms in the body that prioritize homeostasis: *what can get us back to normal as quickly as possible?* It's a nice thought for major stresses like running for your life—who needs to remember to-do lists or lose belly weight when a sabertooth tiger is after you? But for our day-to-day "threats," chronic stress response does nothing for our survival. Instead, we find ourselves trapped in a loop of stress, coping with it in unhealthy ways, becoming too unhealthy to break free, then feeling more stressed than ever.

For example, you might have used the term "stress weight" before. It's true that cortisol tells your body to store fat and not burn in—a remnant of those tiger-chasing days when we needed it for survival. But there's more to stress weight than hormonal shifts. In fact, at least one study suggests that the weight-gain effects of cortisol can be kept at bay with a good diet.(Roberts, et al, 2013) Yet there's a reason carbs and sugars are considered "comfort foods." When we turn to them in times of stress, the immediate dulling of anxiousness and perkup during exhaustion makes us want more. The cortisol wants more and more sugar and carb to turn into fat for storage, and the scale, our waistlines, and our ultimately compromised health wind up paying for it.

It's not just hormones that respond to stress, either; the immune and inflammatory response shifts, and brain pathways fundamentally (meant to be temporarily) change. (For more on the inner workings of the stress response, read *The Balance Within*, by Esther M. Sternberg.) As stress and anxiety build and continue uninhibited, however, researchers have found that these temporary shifts can lead to permanent alteration, including cognitive problems and even dementia. (Mah, et al, 2016)

Entire volumes have been written on the inner workings that get us through tough times. As people in pursuit of a mindset of wellness and life, our concern doesn't lie in things we can't control. Instead, the 5 Essentials seek to eliminate the everyday interference—such as stress-eating—that inhibits or tarnishes those innate functions.

Sleep is Non-Negotiable

Sometimes, a lack of sleep makes us feel stressed. Maybe we've let the daily schedule take over, bombarded with the things everyone needs and the commitments we've made. Or maybe we're going to bed but there's something keeping us from sleeping well. Reflux, apnea, restless leg—going to bed doesn't always mean resting thoroughly.

Adults under the age of 60 should be sleeping at least seven full hours every night. According to the CDC's collection of data, sleeping less than that "is associated with increased risk for obesity, diabetes, high blood pressure, coronary heart disease, stroke, frequent mental distress, and all-cause mortality"—but about 35% of a survey of nearly half a million people don't hit the mark. (Liu, et al, 2016) The more stressful factors in the participant's life, such as being unemployed, the more likely they were to sleep poorly.

Whether sleep becomes difficult because of stressful circumstances or because stress interrupts sleep, the cycle will be difficult to break. Sleep deprivation is connected with cortisol increases and a heightened adrenal response. (Minkel, et al, 2016) Hormones guided by the adrenals are meant to be triggered quickly, then act slowly. When we trigger them consistently, the response can burn out—

leaving us *feeling* burned out. Eventually, the stress response itself will become unregulated and unchecked. Another study of stress and sleep indicated that poor sleep conditions, including night-waking and low quality sleep, lead to poor "cognitive, affective, and physiological responses to stress." (Williams, et al, 2013)

Our bodies simply can't handle stress, reign in a mindset for life, or successfully pursue any of the 5 Essentials without sleep.

You probably know from experience that it's difficult to become motivated to exercise without a good night's rest. When morning comes, you're reaching for coffee, by afternoon you're hoping for a nap, and then you're kicking back on the couch at the end of the day. If you can somehow get outside to walk or build a few minutes of HIIT into that sleepy day, however, you'll probably sleep even better that night. Sleep and exercise are deeply interconnected. (Chennaoui, et al, 2015) Keeping your exercise routine can induce better sleep, and missing out on sleep will undoubtedly make exercise a difficult habit to maintain.

Similarly, as we've already looked at with stress-eating, the way our bodies use food can be directly connected to sleep duration and quality. When we lay down to sleep, it's not only the mind recharging but every cell and process within the body. Food is digested, nutrients are distributed, toxins are eliminated, hormones are regulated, and glucose is mediated. In a recent study, researchers found that chronic sleep deprivation (less than five hours each night) could be a risk factor in the development of type 2 diabetes. (Al-Abri, et al, 2016) So even if you aren't stress-eating—even if you have been trying to follow the Core Nutrition Plan—if you neglect to take care of your mind and body with good, consistent sleep, the nutrients might not be used well anyway.

Think of it this way: You're actually not healing *while* you're drinking that smoothie or *while* you're doing that surge workout or receiving an adjustment. Your body does the related healing when you're *at rest.*

Sleep is simply not negotiable.

Perhaps most importantly—certainly most specific to this aspect of the 5 Essentials—the sleep that we get (or don't get) has a direct impact on our mindset. From normal levels of patience and perspective, to risks of more serious concerns like anxiety and depression, we need consistent sleep habits in order to foster healthy thought patterns. The longer someone is deprived of sleep, the more likely they are to become anxious. (Pires, et al, 2016) If stress is slowly wearing down our bodies, sleep deprivation is wearing down our minds, creating room for more stress, interference, and illness.

Prioritize the Practical

When mindset is discussed, usually it's in terms of the mystical: how to meditate, what to visualize, or which mantras to use. To be sure, those sorts of things can be excellent tools to help you remove mental blocks and free your limited beliefs. But the mind and body aren't separate. As we've already seen, everything is interconnected, sometimes to the extent that you can't tell which came first.

Sometimes, when we're exhausted, stressed out, and in poor health, sitting in a meditative state can feel impractical and impossible to achieve. Where do you find the time? How do you keep from nodding off in an unplanned daytime nap? How can you remember a mantra—or perhaps, from a religious perspective, be rooted in prayer—when your mind is running with *"where did I leave my keys?"*

Throughout this book, the goal has been to empower you to affect real change in your life. Not another list of obligations or self-guided prescriptions, but a framework that you can tailor to your own unique body, life, and family to help bring the innate back into focus. Only you know what's in your way. Only you can remove it and move toward health. In that vein, instead of starting with an exercise or affirmation that will universally bring everyone's mindset into focus (hint: that doesn't exist), we must first begin with the habits and routines that interfere with a healthy mindset in the first place.

Sleep Habits

We spent a lot of time talking about the ills of too little sleep, but good sleep habits should keep you from sleeping too long, as well. Cognitive problems and physical problems alike are connected to all sorts of sleep abnormalities, including sleeping too little *and* sleeping too much. (Bin, Marshall, Glozier, 2013) Cultivating better sleep routines involves consistent times, quality, and duration and sleep. Addressing any underlying health issues is important for sleep quality. Apnea and snoring problems can keep you from resting, even if you feel like you're sleeping. Pain and discomfort can also disrupt sleep quality, though you're likely to know whether that's the case! Don't ever settle. Poor sleep isn't something you put up with or tough your way through.

Similarly, sleep isn't the last thing on the day's list that can be moved around and put off. Don't think of sleep as coming last. When a new day ticks over at 12:00 A.M., what's the first thing you'll be doing that day? Sleeping, hopefully! Think of sleep as the thing that starts your day well—nothing else can have higher priority than sleep. If you've got too much on your plate to manage seven solid hours, you've got too much on your plate.

We've all got the same amount of hours in a day. We all need sleep, and it will catch up with everyone eventually. No one is ever truly at an advantage when burning the candle at both ends. **Seven to eight hours of sleep is not only the ideal duration, but necessary.** Make it your priority.

Routines are the most practical way to stabilize not only sleep but your mindset as a whole. The mechanism that allows someone to grow sleepy in the evening and fall asleep at night, then wake with the sun, is the circadian rhythm. The idea of a rhythm driving your body and guiding you is beautiful—a steady constant that exists beneath all of the music of your day. When routine feels dull or overwhelming, think instead of creating a rhythm that shapes your day, making the most of waking hours and sleeping hours alike.

Regulated Screen Time

Regular waking times, meals, exercise, time in the sun and with your family—the familiarity, consistency, and connection all contribute to that sense of rhythm and routine that puts our minds at ease, allowing us to rest. But there's also a much more utilitarian, unappealing, unattractive change we can make to set our internal clock back on track: cut the evening screen time.

Put down the cell phone once you're in bed, at minimum. Hours before bed, set the screen to an amber tone and dial down the brightness. Get an actual clock by your bedside and store the phone in the nightstand to break the habit of middle-of-the-night looks at the clock on your home screen. Why? The contrast and blue tint of a cell phone light stands in stark opposition to the warm, fading light of a sunset into darkness.

Our bodies can't be tricked into accepting blue light as a signal of impending sleep. Instead, we have to change our routines or the light that hits our eyes. One of the more recent studies on screen time and sleep found that amber lenses instead of clear lenses at night—two hours before bedtime—helped people with insomnia to sleep better. (Shechter, 2018) Another study in adolescents noted the particular sensitivity that kid have to screen time. Melatonin levels—the internal function that triggers sleepiness as daylight fades in the evening—dropped by 23 and 38 percent with one or two hours of screen time, respectively. (Figueiro, Overington, 2016)

Most phones and tablets have settings that change the tone of the screen from harsh blue and white toned lights to sepia or amber color schemes. Better yet, turn the TV off and tuck the screens away before bed, choosing instead to calm and relax your body in preparation for sleep. You can cover up any digital clocks in your bedroom to tone down the digital light in the room, as well.

It's not just sleep that's disrupted by screens, either. Screen times, including computers and TV, in excess of six hours per day can be a predictor of depression, especially for women. (Madhav, Sherchand, Sherchan, 2017) Again, whether it's the cause or a response isn't clear and doesn't matter. A clear mind and healthy focus exist best when we're interacting with nature (and one another) more than screens, lights, and keys.

Essential Focus

The brain is often compared to a computer, but mindset goes even deeper than that. If the body were a machine, the mind would be not only the computer but the hard-drive and software. It affects the way the systems are run. By the same token, a flaw in the system will affect the way it works, as well. So while we have to allow the body and mind to rest in order to pursue the other aspects of the 5 Essentials effectively, we also have to pursue the 5 Essentials in order to have a healthy mindset.

Many of the professions that are labeled complementary and alternative medicine alongside chiropractic—though we don't necessarily claim that label—are sought after because of their stress-relieving, relaxing, whole-body effects. In Core Chiropractic, we looked at the way a stressed body can hold tension and interference in the spine. As chiropractors, we see people every day who come in for discomfort or who are simply interested in better alignment, then come back regularly because they simply *feel* better. Not just structurally, but as a matter of mindset. When the spine is stressed, the nervous system is stressed, and that impacts both the body and the mind. It's why a growing number of people making chiropractic care part of their regular routine on a preventive basis.

Within the Core and Advanced Nutrition Plans, we took a deep dive into the way food affect us—what our bodies expect to utilize and how they cope when we fill up on other things. The connection between diet and mood is self-evident. Comfort foods seem to soothe the mind, but in reality they are keeping us from digesting well, using food energy well, and even affecting the way we sleep. (Grandner, et al, 2014) When our brains are fed with good, nourishing fats, and the foods we eat provide nutrients that feed and restore our bodies from a cellular level, we feel more rested, stabilized, and happy.

In our focus on exercise, we looked to bursts of high intensity effort to keep our muscles—including heart and lungs—strong but not stressed. Oxygen as part of that essential, and toxin elimination as the next, are also meant to keep oxygen and nutrients circulated through the body while scavenging for toxins. Deep, focused breathing meets both of those needs, feeding the body and removing at least some toxicants from our cells. Calming movement practices like yoga, tai chi, and meditation sessions can teach us to fill our lungs, breathe through the moment, and move our bodies and minds in careful, synchronized flows. (Bankar, Chaudhari, 2013) Better breath control—especially when practiced in fresh air— trains our lungs to expel more, eliminating more of the inevitable toxins and pollutants in the environment.

A Perspective for Life

All facets of MaxLiving are interconnected. As we take steps toward health in one area of our lives, the effects ripple throughout others that we might not even be aware of. Sometimes we can spot the interference that should be removed but have no grasp on the benefits that will follow. Sometimes it takes awhile to identify the interference, so we keep doing the next right thing no matter what tangible results there may or may not be.

Though we can never set the practical steps completely aside, neither can we ignore the importance of a positive, healthy outlook. It's a step beyond or outside of medicine—we aren't here just to fix things that are wrong. We are here to gain a new perspective on what it means to be healthy. A new, proactive perspective on—and of and for—life.

Mindfulness

The very idea of the innate, if you step back and envision it in action, is incredible. **The capabilities that lie within us are far greater than our limiting beliefs tell us.** We have one chance at this life, and it was not meant to grow complacent in pain, discomfort, and depression, though many of us will find some of those things are part of our lives—complete absence of disease is not always a realistic expectation. It's our approach, our mindset that makes the difference. Allowing ourselves to marvel at the design of the human body is motivation in itself to remove all interference that holds us back from mitigating those diseases and misfortunes as they arise.

Mindfulness as a practice asks us to do just that. To acknowledge the moment we are in—circumstances, feelings, thoughts, obstacles, and potential—and nothing more. There's a time for planning and moving forward, of course, and through the 5 Essentials, we've covered many (though not all) of the ways that you can. But mindfulness asks us to just sit with the moment we're in, if only for a little while. You can't change what it was that brought you here, and you can't control what will come tomorrow. But you can appreciate, accept, and admire the intricacies of *self* that exist in this moment.

The practice of mindfulness has shown itself to be viable—at times, exceptional—for many of our daily stressors, big and small. In the workplace, for example, mindfulness practices can be used to reduce stress in employees and the office as a whole. (Arredondo, 2017) A review of an extensive database of studies tells us that mindfulness can be an effective tool to use when struggling with depression, pain, and addiction. (Goldberg, S. B., et al, 2018) There are implications for sleep, stress, physical and mental health, elderly, students, and more.

Try this: **Take a few moments to do nothing but breathe.** Then take a few more to focus on breathing deeper. Then, keep breathing as you roll your neck around and loosen your shoulders. Wiggle fingers, shift your hips and settle them into your seat. Shake your thighs loose, and roll your feet around at your ankles. Each step of the way, keep the focus on your breath and that area of your body. Not to judge quality or add to your list of aches and pains, but only to *notice*. Acknowledge where there might be tension, accept it for what it is, and move on. Finally, sit for a moment with your thoughts. Allow them to come and go, only noticing them (as you did with the rest of your body.)

After you've spent a few minutes here—five is plenty, especially when you're just starting out—simply continue on with the rest of your day. Mindfulness and, truly, a maximized mindset only asks us to be present with our thoughts and our bodies. Our world is compartmentalized. Over time, our bodies and minds become disjointed. Reconnecting them through mindfulness and awareness helps to lay the foundation of an outlook of health—an innate perspective.

Gratitude and Joy

Underlying all of the practical steps toward a healthier mindset, a sense of gratitude and joy become the real drivers. As you learn to relax, prioritize sleep, and shake off stressful situations, it becomes easier to find a sense of peace than when you've got your head down, running the rat race. Or—more likely—if you're struggling to get a handle on the practical, consider starting slowly, but more profoundly, with your perspective.

If you were to strip away all pretense to be completely honest, how do you truly feel about your life? Sure, we're supposed to say we're grateful, but if you dig deeper than the cursory smiles and sense of obligation, you might find something closer to the truth. Society tells us to never be satisfied, always finding flaws and pressing for more. To some extent, it's good to strive for the best. But marketing departments don't want us to *actually* find or become the best, or to be content with the slow journey. It's easy enough to mask discontent under the façade of self help, even the pursuit of the 5 Essentials. But that's not how this truly works.

An extensive survey of Swedish adults found that not only is gratitude associated with better health, but better health habits as well. (Hill, Allemand, Roberts, 2013) People who expressed a sense of gratitude and contentment, enjoying their life in the moment for what it was, were more likely to treat their bodies well. They exercised more, ate better, and sought help when they needed it. **Gratitude is not the same as complacency.** Instead, gratitude honors and appreciates our bodies and our lives, implicitly. There's less guilt and shame in a grateful life, fewer "shoulds" that keep driving us toward someone else's expectations. Not only does that shake off a good bit of stress, but it also builds an appreciation for our bodies that can motivate us toward better habits and practical steps.

Today's motivational gurus may have you striving for big goals and "what's next." I'll add one caveat. If you want to get there with any sense of joy—which I believe is paramount— you've got to be happy where you are *right now.*

A life of gratitude is marked by contentedness and peace; a life of joy might be identified by laughter. How often do you laugh each day? How hard are you laughing when you do? If it's difficult to answer that question, you're not alone. We all go through times of trouble or reservation, all too easily caught up in our own thoughts and worries. But when Japanese researchers evaluated survey responses of over 20,000 people, they found that people who laughed more had better health. (Hayashi, et al, 2016)

Even after accounting for all other factors, there was no other apparent explanation but that people who laughed every day had better cardiovascular health and less risk of stroke. **Laughter may well be the best medicine, and it's best delivered with gratefulness, joy, and meaningful human connection.**

Maximized Mindset

We keep eating well even when we haven't lost weight right away. We exercise even when our pants size stays the same. We rid our homes clear of toxic products, even when "we've always done it" a certain way. We visit the chiropractor even when we are not symptomatic. This is a radical departure from the prevailing perspectives in our society. It's not prescriptive. It's not reactive. It's a proactive choice to do what we know our bodies need, regardless of any immediate benefit.

Gratitude walks hand in hand with joy, and both are correlated with connections to friends, family, community, and our own selves. If screen time is making us depressed, the antidote may simply be connection with people rather than the curated images of people that social media or marketing teams want us to see. There is a deep-seated joy that can only be found in community, leading us back to the World Health Organization's definition of health, including "social well-being" as one of several pillars.

In spite of the time-tried ideal of complete health from the inside out, world health has arguably moved away from that wisdom in recent decades. For our purposes—as practitioners, teachers, leaders, parents, people—that's okay. We can't change the whole world all at once, and we don't have to. We have each other. We have ourselves. One by one, taking whatever steps we can, changing whatever thoughts and beliefs we can, our own view of health will change. Ultimately, the way we manage health will change. And then we will change. Eventually, the world *will* change—but it all begins with these first, essential steps.

25 Books Simplified by 5 Essentials

Larry Shaw

"

Once I was diagnosed with Type 2 diabetes, my doctor started me on Metformin to manage my blood sugar levels. Over the next few years, my doctor altered my medications because some became ineffective and others created side effects. In fact, most of the medications I took worsened my diabetes. I felt like I was in a vicious cycle.

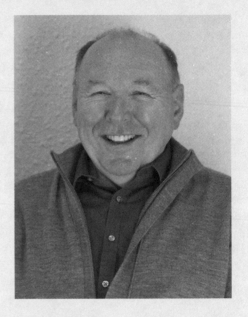

About a year after I was diagnosed, I attended a MaxLiving seminar. I subsequently read the book put out by MaxLiving about its nutrition plan.

Before starting anything, I wanted to process things. There is no doubt that I was skeptical. After all, I had read about twenty-five other books and felt a lot of doubt that food and lifestyle could really do me or my diabetes any good. Regardless, that following New Year's Day, I committed to follow the Advanced Plan.

The first three weeks on the program were the most difficult, but things fell into place. About a month after I began, I started feeling better. The first thing I noticed is that I felt about twenty-five years younger on this program. Then, the weight loss benefits were secondary.

As for my diabetes, my blood sugar levels began to stabilize. Over time, my doctor gradually tapered me off my medications. Eventually, I was able to go off other medications my doctor had prescribed, including those for high cholesterol and high blood pressure. Even my sleep improved.

Altogether, I've lost about eighty pounds. I've learned from MaxLiving that the best medicine—at least for me—is real food. Through some simple dietary changes, I've reversed diabetes, lost weight, and now feel so much better. I know I've also reduced my risk for other diseases. My immune system also improved; I no longer get seasonal flus and colds. Should I get a sniffle today, a good night's sleep is usually all I need to feel better.

I can now work more effectively than ever before. I'm able to stay more focused. I get seven to eight hours of solid, deep sleep almost every night. My knees and other joints feel much better. I am back to playing sports regularly. My cognitive and emotional health have greatly improved, I am back to learning new things and almost nothing bothers me like it used to.

Today, when issues come my way, I immediately look for solutions rather than focus on the problems.

I went to my doctor about a week ago to review my blood work. I had not seen him for two years, and my weight was the same as the previous visit. My blood pressure was good and my A1C was in the range of a non-diabetic person. My doctor said that if I were a new patient, he would not consider me diabetic.

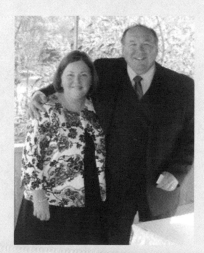

BEFORE

I am completely off all medications. I focus on eating local, organic, and real food. I avoid packaged foods and foods filled with chemicals. This plan has truly changed my health and my life forever.

It's changed my wife's life, too. (She's lost 120 lbs.)

Part Three

Appendices

Appendix A
Core Plan Food Guide

Appendix B
Advanced Plan Food Guide

Appendix C
Navigating the Grocery Store

Appendix D
Kitchen Essentials

Appendix E
Simple Swaps for Everyday Life

Appendix F
Quick Reference Exercise Guide

Appendix G
Meal Planning for Success

APPENDICES
Making it Work

Whether you're finishing a cover-to-cover read or flipping to the sections that help you out right now, you've taken in a lot of information. The last thing I want to do is to blend into the noise of every other do-and-don't list out there. I want you to take what you've learned and are learning here and feel empowered to apply it to the framework of your own life.

In the hierarchy of undesirable options, the worst thing you can do with this information is to get overwhelmed and not prioritize anything. I've given you the knowledge; now, I want to leave you with some of the tools you'll need to apply it.

I fully respect and acknowledge that some organic, non-GMO foods can still contain problematic chemicals. I further respect that, to this day, there are a lack of human studies demonstrating better health as a result of going organic. But what we do know is enough for me—and we all must do the best we can with what we have. This really comes down to two things: what you will accept as a matter of principle, and what you can realistically begin to prioritize for the sake of better health and fuller lives.

Again, we aren't looking at things that cause immediate illness or keep us from "turning out fine." We're concerned with the slow accumulation of interference, from all sources, that build up over time and lead to major health concerns, and children are at a great deal of risk in that regard. There are simply more years left in their lives for all of these things to accumulate. But that also means they have more years left to correct, and the sooner we can help our children make good decisions, the better off they will be as adults.

So in the midst of your busy life—fast-paced schedules and so much on your plate, not to mention picky eaters and tight budgets—how can you take what you've learned and apply it to your life and your household?

1. Baby steps

The best first-steps you can take are the steps that will stick. If you can change the kinds of meats you buy, but you can't give up that instant breakfast yet, do it! If you need to follow the Dirty Dozen instead of going completely organic, then enjoy your conventional oranges and organic apples! We're in this for the long haul, and every step you take toward a healthier family is a good one.

2. Do it together

Work together with friends, as a couple, or with your kids to implement the 5 Essentials. Do your surge cycles together. Make a meal plan that everyone contributes to. Pick a couple of new recipes and have a "potluck" with your friends. Cook with your kids. Go on a mindfulness walk together, and then talk about the things you observed and experienced. Social health is as important to this process as anything, so don't go it alone!

3. Keep at it

It's going to take some time to settle in. That's why we don't ask you to do everything at once. If you're like most of us, you have years or decades or a lifetime of habits and cycles to undo. It'll take some time for your brain to adjust to this new lifestyle map, and that's okay. You need lots of repetition to make this second nature. Keep doing it, even when you "fall off the wagon." Kids need lots of exposure to new foods before they can trust and enjoy them. Keep presenting it to them, letting them taste, see, and get used to it as a new normal slowly, over time.

This is a process. Be good to yourself, your family, and your world throughout it. Keep reading through the appendix for more tips, tools, and resources to help you along the way.

APPENDIX A

The Core Nutrition Plan

Our nutrition plans don't count calories or assign rigid portion sizes. Remember, our goal is to get reacquainted with Innate Intelligence and what our bodies need. In order to remove nutritional interference and get back to that place of dietary wellness, follow the Core Nutrition Plan.

Fat	Protein	Carbohydrates
Eat more healthy fats. Eliminate all damaged fats.	If consuming animal protein, always select from organic & naturally-raised sources.	Eat more vegetables. Eliminate refined grains and sugars.

Remember:

- Choose organic whenever possible.
- Consume any higher sugar plant-based foods earlier in the day.
- Enjoy a variety of options in every meal, and eat until you're full.

How to use this list

Choose foods from the categories listed based on the quality requirements described. Examples are given, and the Grocery Store Cheat Sheet (Appendix C) can help you get started. If you discover new favorites that meet the requirements, eat up! If you find that you don't tolerate some foods well or thrive as a vegetarian, adapt as necessary. When in doubt, revisit chapter four.

This is not a diet—it's a lifestyle of wellness and a better relationship with food.

Plant-Based Carbohydrates

Avoid pesticides and GMO crops. If fat burning is a priority, consume moderate-sugar options before lunch only and avoid higher-sugar carbohydrates altogether until you stabilize.

Vegetables		
High-fiber, low-sugar vegetables are your best carbohydrate choices, any time of the day.		
Arugula	Asparagus	Bamboo shoots
Bean sprouts	Bell pepper	Broad beans
Broccoli	Brussels sprouts	Cabbage
Cauliflower	Chives	Celery
Chayote fruit	Chicory	Coriander
Collard greens	Cucumber	Eggplant
Endive	Fennel	Garlic
Ginger root	Green beans	Hearts of palm
Jicama	Jalapeño peppers	Kale
Kohlrabi	Lettuce	Mushrooms
Parsley	Mustard greens	Onions
Radishes	Radicchio	Snap beans
Snow peas	Shallots	Spinach
Spaghetti squash	Summer squash	Swiss chard
Tomatoes	Turnip greens	Watercress
Zucchini		

Plant-Based Carbohydrates – *continued*

Low-sugar fruits		
Low-sugar fruits are tolerated well throughout the day. Include more earlier in the day.		
Granny Smith apple	Lemon	Limes
Berries		
Blackberries	Blueberries	Boysenberries
Elderberries	Gooseberries	Loganberries
Raspberries	Strawberries	

Moderate-sugar fruits		
Consume in moderation, no later than lunchtime.		
Apples	Apricots	Cherries
Grapefruit	Kiwi	Melon
Nectarines	Oranges	Passion fruit
Peaches	Pears	Persimmons
Plums	Pomegranate	Prunes
Tangerines		

Higher-sugar fruits		
Consume in small portions only and earlier in the day. These are best consumed on high-activity days and post-exercise.		
Bananas	Dates	Grapes
Mango	Papaya	Pineapple
Watermelon		

Plant-Based Carbohydrates – *continued*

Legumes, tubers, and root vegetables		
Consume in moderation and earlier in the day. These carbohydrates are balanced in fiber and sugar and can be eliminated altogether if fat burning is a priority.		
Artichoke	Adzuki beans	Beets
Black beans	Carrots	Cassava
Chickpeas (garbanzo)	Cowpeas	French beans
Great Northern beans	Kidney beans	Leeks
Lentils	Lima beans	Mung beans
Navy beans	Okra	Pinto beans
Pumpkin	Split peas	Sweet potato/yam
Tapioca	White beans	Yellow beans

Grains		
Emphasize ancient grains, pseudograins and non-gluten grains. "Enriched" denotes a food product that has been stripped of its naturally occurring nutrients and replenished with vitamins afterward. Food in its whole form is always preferable. Always consume whole, sprouted and stone-ground versions. Avoid after lunchtime.		
Ancient grains & pseudograins		
Amaranth	Buckwheat	Farro*
Kamut*	Millet	Quinoa
Sorghum	Spelt*	Teff
Whole grains		
Barley*	Brown rice	Oats
Rye*	Wheat*	Wild rice
* Avoid if gluten is a concern. Note: Oats are by nature gluten-free, but often contaminated.		

Healthy Fats & Proteins

Prioritize low-to-no processing, avoid oil rancidity, and avoid secondary toxin exposure through animal proteins raised conventionally.

Nuts & seeds		
Almonds	Cashews	Chia seeds
Flax seeds	Hemp seeds	Macadamia
Pecans	Pine nuts	Pumpkin seeds
Sesame seeds	Sunflower seeds	Walnuts

Raw nut & seed butter		
Almond butter	Cashew butter	Macadamia butter
Pumpkin seed butter	Raw tahini	

Coconut		
Coconut butter	Coconut chips	Coconut flour
Coconut meat	Coconut milk	

Oils		
Avocado oil *	Cod liver oil	Extra virgin coconut oil *
Extra virgin olive oil *	Flaxseed oil	Hemp seed oil
Walnut oil		
* These oils can be heated, provided they do not smoke. Others should never be heated.		

Fermented soy		
Miso	Tempeh	Tamari

Healthy Fats & Proteins – *continued*

Animal proteins		
Chicken	Eggs	Grass-fed beef
Lamb	Turkey	Wild fish*
Any animal products should be organic and sustainably-raised.		
* Always select wild fish from clean waters (best examples are Pacific and Alaskan salmon, Mahi-mahi, halibut) with an emphasis on small fish (sardines, anchovies).		

Dairy		
Use caution with dairy. Choose full fat, organic dairy at a bare minimum. Non-homogenized dairy is even better. Unpasteurized (raw) and A2 dairy are most ideal, when available from a trusted source.		
Butter	Cream	Ghee
Kefir	Raw cheese	Yogurt

If you have followed the Core Nutrition Plan and still find yourself feeling unwell, consider eliminating common irritants. Dairy and gluten are common culprits— but, use caution with special dairy-free and gluten-free products, as they can be loaded with sugar, preservatives and more. At first, it's easier to eliminate than it is to replace! Enjoy simple preparations of sprouted and gluten-free grains and plenty of vegetables while you slowly learn to make or source grain-free and gluten-free breads and crackers.

APPENDIX B

The Advanced Nutrition Plan

We usually turn to the Advanced Nutrition Plan in short-term situations— management of weight, minimal interference during disease or detoxification, and added support for cognitive, metabolic, and immune health—though some people can certainly thrive on it for the longer term.

The goal is to reduce the consumption of inflammatory foods, nourish the body on a cellular level, support regular hormone function, and promote the use of fat (instead of sugar) as the body's primary source for energy. It works well, and it works fast.

Here are some indicators you may wish to follow this plan:

- Blood sugar irregularities
- Heart disease or metabolic syndrome:
  ○ Blood pressure irregularities
  ○ High cholesterol
  ○ High triglycerides
- Hormonal imbalances
- Obesity or weight-loss resistance
- Systemic or local inflammation
- Digestive dysfunction
- Immune challenges (autoimmunity, low immunity, cancer)
- Cognitive stress or disorders (Autism spectrum disorders, ADD/ADHD, mood or sleep imbalances)
- Chronic fatigue, fibromyalgia

Fat	Protein	Carbohydrates
Eat more healthy fats. Eliminate all damaged fats.	Moderate your intake of protein.	Eliminate grains, most fruit, and all sugar.

Remember these guidelines when you begin the Advanced Nutrition Plan:

- Organic, non-processed, non-GMO choices are vital.
- Don't start slow—plan well and jump in all at once.
- Expect to struggle with cravings and difficulty adjusting for the first two weeks, though almost everyone settles in after that.

How to use this list

The Advanced Nutrition Plan has more specific goals within each macronutrient group. Pay close attention to the guidelines for each, and again, enjoy nourishing options until you're satisfied. When in doubt, revisit chapter four.

Plant-Based Carbohydrates

As always, avoid pesticides and GMO crops. Higher-sugar fruits and all grains are eliminated on the Advanced Plan due to their impact on insulin and on inflammation.

Vegetables		
High-fiber, low-sugar vegetables are your best carbohydrate choices, any time of the day.		
Arugula	Asparagus	Bamboo shoots
Bean sprouts	Bell peppers	Broad beans
Broccoli	Brussels sprouts	Cabbage
Cauliflower	Chives	Celery
Chayote fruit	Chicory	Coriander
Collard greens	Cucumber	Eggplant
Endive	Fennel	Garlic
Ginger root	Green beans	Hearts of palm
Jicama	Jalapeño peppers	Kale
Kohlrabi	Lettuce	Mushrooms
Parsley	Mustard greens	Onions
Radishes	Radicchio	Snap beans
Snow peas	Shallots	Spinach
Spaghetti squash	Summer squash	Swiss chard
Tomatoes	Turnip greens	Watercress
Zucchini		

Plant-Based Carbohydrates – *continued*

Low-sugar fruits		
Low-sugar fruits are tolerated well throughout the day. Include more earlier in the day.		
Granny Smith apple	Lemon	Limes
Berries		
Blackberries	Blueberries	Boysenberries
Elderberries	Gooseberries	Loganberries
Raspberries	Strawberries	

Legumes, tubers, and root vegetables		
Consume minimally, and not on a daily basis.		
Artichoke	Adzuki beans	Beets
Black beans	Carrots	Cassava
Chickpeas (garbanzo)	Cowpeas	French beans
Great Northern beans	Kidney beans	Leeks
Lentils	Lima beans	Mung beans
Navy beans	Okra	Pinto beans
Pumpkin	Split peas	Sweet potato/yam
Tapioca	White beans	Yellow beans

Healthy Fats & Proteins

Prioritize low-to-no processing, avoid oil rancidity, and avoid secondary toxin exposure through animal proteins raised conventionally.

Nuts & seeds		
Almonds	Cashews	Chia seeds
Flax seeds	Hemp seeds	Macadamia
Pecans	Pine nuts	Pumpkin seeds
Sesame seeds	Sunflower seeds	Walnuts

Raw nut & seed butter		
Almond butter	Cashew butter	Macadamia butter
Pumpkin seed butter	Raw tahini	

Coconut		
Coconut butter	Coconut chips	Coconut flour
Coconut meat	Coconut milk	

Oils		
Avocado oil *	Cod liver oil	Extra virgin coconut oil *
Extra virgin olive oil *	Flaxseed oil	Hemp seed oil
Walnut oil		
* These oils can be heated, provided they do not smoke. Others should never be heated.		

Fermented soy		
Miso	Tempeh	Tamari

Healthy Fats & Proteins – *continued*

Animal proteins		
Chicken	Eggs	Grass-fed beef
Lamb	Turkey	Wild fish*
Any animal products should be organic and sustainably-raised.		
* Always select wild fish from clean waters (best examples are Pacific and Alaskan salmon, Mahi-mahi, halibut) with an emphasis on small fish (sardines, anchovies).		

Dairy		
On the Advanced Plan, extra caution should be exercised with dairy. Even the most optimal dairy choices can be inflammatory and affect insulin levels. Asalways,, when incorporating any dairy products, choose full fat, organic dairy at a bare minimum. Non-homogenized dairy is even better. Unpasteurized (raw) and A2 dairy are most ideal, when available from a trusted source.		
Butter	Cream	Ghee
Kefir	Raw cheese	Yogurt

APPENDIX C

Navigating the Grocery Store

Every year, the Environmental Working Group releases a list of the Dirty Dozen and Clean Fifteen produce choices, detailing the 12 most important fruits and vegetables to buy organic and 15 options that can be safe when grown conventionally. The 2017 list reveals the following:

Dirty Dozen+		
Always buy organic.		
Strawberries	Spinach	Nectarines
Apples	Peaches	Pears
Cherries	Grapes	Celery
Tomatoes	Sweet bell peppers	Potatoes
Hot peppers		

Clean Fifteen		
If budget is a concern, you can purchase the following types of conventional produce:		
Sweet corn	Avocados	Pineapples
Cabbage	Onions	Sweet peas (frozen)
Papayas	Asparagus	Mangos
Eggplant	Honeydew melon	Kiwi
Cantaloupe	Cauliflower	Grapefruit

Dodging GMOs

Selecting conventional vs. organic produce based solely on the EWG guide to the Clean Fifteen and Dirty Dozen could be problematic if you are aiming to avoid GMOs, as well.

Though sweet corn and papaya are on the Clean Fifteen for pesticide concentration, some sweet corn and papaya sold in North America is produced from genetically modified seeds.

Buy organic varieties of the following Core Plan and Advanced Plan crops if you want to avoid GMO produce:

- Alfalfa
- Papaya
- Yellow squash and zucchini
- Sugar beet

While corn, canola, and soy are also largely genetically modified, you need not worry as these foods are neither on the Core Plan or the Advanced Plan, for other reasons. Fermented soy such as miso, tempeh and tamari may be acceptable; look for an emphasis on the label that it is non-GMO when buying it.

Seafood Shopping

The Monterey Bay Aquarium Seafood Watch produces regularly-updated, science-based and region-by-region consumer guides to help consumers and businesses make healthy seafood choices. Their "best" choices are fish to buy first; they are well managed and caught or farmed responsibly. The "good alternatives" raise some concern with how they are farmed or caught. The "avoid" list covers seafoods that are overfished or caught/farmed in ways that harm other marine life or the environment. Download a guide via www.seafoodwatch.org.

Some farmed options may appear on your local guide. The MaxLiving approach would urge you to select wild-caught and smaller fish from clean waters that also receive an endorsement from Seafood Watch.

Selecting Sweeteners

Simple sugars		
Avoid completely when added to foods in their elemental forms.		
Sugar	Brown sugar	Fructose
Glucose	Dextrose	Sucanat
Cornstarch	Corn sugar	

Syrups and saps		
Avoid at all costs. These liquids are made up of nearly 100% simple sugars and all will increase the glycemic and caloric loads of foods, in varying degrees.		
Agave nectar or syrup	Coconut nectar or syrup	Cane syrup or cane juice
Molasses	Corn syrup and high-fructose corn syrup	
Grade B maple syrup*	Raw honey*	

* Raw, undenatured honey and Grade B maple syrup are the least-processed options in this category and, therefore, would be considered the most "whole" forms of sugar on this list. Some individuals may metabolize these as unrefined foods easier than other refined sugars on our lists. But, neither are considered substitutes for simple sugar on the Core Plan or Advanced Plan but could be used minimally in desserts or beverages when breaking from the MaxLiving Plan, while remaining as true to its principles, as possible. Honey, though it possesses medicinal properties, is still 99% sugar and maple syrup can offer a sizeable glycemic load to your body.

Chemically-processed, artificial sweeteners
Avoid entirely.
Aspartame (Equal, NutraSweet, Candarel)
Sucralose (Splenda, Zerocal, Sukrana, SucraPlus, Candys, Cukren, Nevella)

Selecting Sweeteners – *continued*

Whole food origins		
Whole fruits, though some are higher in sugar than others, are your best options for sweetening foods you make yourself or buy at the store.		
Banana puree	Whole apple sauce	Pure fruit juice*
Whole dried fruits, including dates*		
* Exercise caution with dried fruits, particularly dates, as these can affect insulin levels more substantially than can whole, undried fruits. Fruit juice is acceptable in very minimal amounts although, depending on the recipe, you're always better off with the entire fruit!		

Plant-based, safer sweeteners		
Stevia	Lakanto	Sugar alcohols*
* Sugar alcohols such as xylitol, maltitol and erythritol can disrupt bacterial flora and cause digestive distress. Use sparingly on any MaxLiving nutrition plan. Erythritol appears to cause problems in the least number of people.		

Stevia Guide

With the market adoption of stevia and the numerous forms that are now available, it is not possible to distinctively always say that there is an exact fraction of extract that would be used "instead of" sugar or spoonable stevia. There is no simple conversion chart. Learn about your options and adjust recipes to your taste. You can cut the new flavor of stevia but still leverage its sweetness by pairing it with vanilla extract, cinnamon, and/or other spices and flavors.

Spoonable Stevia Powder

Typically bulked up with fiber, this type of stevia is manufactured to be used in same quantities as white sugar for recipes calling for sugar in specific amounts. Use caution as some may be bulked up with corn derivatives such as maltodextrin or sugar alcohols. Recipes in this book actually do not use this form of stevia, though this type can be convenient when adding to tea, coffee, applesauce, yogurt, particularly when making a transition from sugar. You may even find packets in coffee shops, or purchase them for easy transport.

Stevia Extract Powder

Stevia extract powder is far more concentrated than spoonable stevia powder. It is therefore much sweeter. Recipes may call for what seems to be a very small amount of stevia, but when it is this form, a small amount is all that you need.

Liquid Stevia Drops

Best used in beverages. Powders might not dissolve in cold beverages like iced tea or lemonade. Some healthy recipes (including some in this book) use liquid stevia—which is still highly concentrated—e.g. sauces, puddings, beverages. Ultimately, the type of stevia you choose depends on the recipe as a whole.

Oil Changes

Purchase oils in small quantities. Keep them away from light and keep them refrigerated when possible to prevent rancidity. The only oils identified with high-enough smoke points for pan-frying include coconut oil and avocado oil.

The further an oil is from being cold-pressed, the more processing it requires—from solvents to unlabeled trans-fat conversion. The term extra virgin denotes the first press.

The MaxLiving plans also lean towards oils with higher Omega 3 ratios with respect to Omega 6 and Omega 9.

Oils to eliminate		
Canola oil	Cottonseed oil	Poppyseed oil
Vegatable oil	Soybean oil	Palm oil
Corn oil	Peanut oil	
Avoid any vegetable oil that isn't extra virgin or cold pressed.		

Oils to moderate		
Certain recipes on the Core and Advanced Plans may turn out best with these oils, which should be used in moderation on only when extra-virgin and cold-pressed. Look for non-GMO options and keep these cold to avoid rancidity. Smoke or browning is an indication of denaturing.		
Sesame oil	Safflower oil	Sunflower oil
Grapeseed oil		

Oils to include		
Extra virgin olive oil	Extra virgin coconut oil	Avocado oil
Walnut oil	Almond oil	Flax oil
Hemp seed oil		

Replacing Salad Dressings

Oil and vinegar are excellent replacements for conventional salad dressings—provided you use the right oils and the right vinegars! Particularly when you are out and about, order any of these with extra virgin olive oil to top your veggie-rich salad:

- Balsamic vinegar
- Apple cider vinegar
- Lemon juice

Remember: Even the healthiest oils should be used sparingly. The whole food form of coconut oil is the coconut and the whole food form of avocado oil is the avocado. Whole foods aren't processed in any fashion and can often be worked into recipes in place of their pressed oils. Although some oils are safer for cooking, you're ultimately safest cooking with water and adding oils in for flavour once the temperature comes down.

Sauces

As you begin to read labels, you will soon realize that most sauces are loaded with sugar and additives that you won't want to consume. In addition to making your own mayonnaises, salsas, barbeque sauce, dressings and other sauces, there are some good options at the grocery store.

- Sugar-free hot sauce
- Fermented tamari
- Coconut liquid aminos

Use with eggs, meats, veggies and as marinades.
Always ensure they are sugar-free and preferably organic.

Beverages

Obviously, we aren't going to endorse sodas or alcoholic beverages mixed with sugars, heavy with wheat, or consumed in quantities that tax your liver. For the grey areas of other beverages, remember to prioritize water above all else. The rule of thumb is half your bodyweight in ounces, per day.

Water		
Pure spring water	Filtered water	Plain sparkling water*
* Sparkling water is known to create some hunger suppression and can keep you satiated between meals.		

Coffee and tea		
Herbal, green, and white teas		
Dark-roast coffee	Swiss Water decaf coffee	
Use caution with coffee. The coffee bean is highly-sprayed with pesticides and should, therefore, always be purchased organic. Remember: what you put in your coffee (conventional dairy, sugar) is likely much worse for you than the actual coffee, but avoid becoming dependent on it. You're in a better state of control to enjoy coffee for its taste, maybe as a treat, than to be reliant upon it. Similarly, with tea, be sure to purchase organic, well-sourced teas. Further minimize toxins by bagging your own loose-leaf teas in non-toxic tea bags or in a loose leaf diffuser.		

Dairy alternatives		
Almond	Cashew	Coconut
Macadamia		
White beverages certainly do not fall into the category of required nutrients, but any of the above can take care of the cultural tendency for "milk." Avoid soy and avoid sweetened options—you can always add stevia, if necessary. Homemade beverages without fillers and preservatives are always best!		

APPENDIX D
Kitchen Essentials

Slow-cooker

Prep your meals the night before, in the morning for dinner, or make and freeze bags of ingredients to toss in and let it cook. Meals cook in 4-8 hours.

Pressure-cooker

Electric pressure-cookers offer a similar "set it and forget it" benefit, but with faster cooking times. Excellent for last minute meals, meats, and fresh vegetables.

Large stock pot

Make veggie-rich soups and your own broth in a tall, deep stock pot. Avoid teflon-based non-stick.

Cast iron skillets, various sizes

Learn to season and care for cast iron skillets, which become non-stick without the problematic residue. Alternate cookware choices include enameled cast iron, stainless steel, ceramic/Thermolon™, and glass. Beware of teflon non-stick, as well as teflon-relatives, including both PFOAs and PFASs.

Food processor

Efficiently chop, shred, and puree vegetables for salads, dips, soups and snacks.

Blender

A great blender can be a substantial investment, but it should last at least a decade, as it will become much more of an appliance than an accessory. Going far beyond smoothies, you'll use your blender for hot and cold soups, sauces, and homemade desserts.

Spiralizer

Spiralize zucchini, squash, and even sweet potato to create noodles ("zoodles") in place of spaghetti or linguine.

Steamer

Steaming vegetables is the healthiest way to cook them. Only 15% of the water-soluble nutrients are lost in steaming, but because you can often increase your overall intake when veggies are steamed, you're not at a net loss.

Food dehydrator

A dehydrator is not an essential, but it will come in handy as you advance your nutrition plan and create varieties of kale chips, fruit leathers, and grain-free crackers. Many of these can be done without a dehydrator or in the oven, but the dehydrator keeps more nutrients intact with more reliable results.

Immersion blender

Another gadget that isn't vital but can be nice. Make dressings, and puree or thicken soups. Even some smoothies can be made with an immersion blender!

Good set of knives

Kitchen prep is so much easier when you can chop, slice, dice, and julienne with ease. Do your whole-foods recipes a favor and invest in a good set of knives. Vital pieces: chef's knife, carving knife, paring knife.

Stainless-steel water bottles

You need to keep water with you wherever you go, and stainless steel bottles provide the best option without risking BPA, broken glass, or spills. Follow cleaning guidelines to avoid rust.

Reusable food storage containers (if plastic, BPA-free)

Preparing and making food ahead of time will make it easier to stay on track, especially during times of travel and busy schedules. Get various sizes to freeze excess soup, pre-make lunches, package leftovers into other recipes, etc.

Non-toxic dish soap

Several brands provide safe dish soap, and castile can always be used, too. Not only are better soaps good for your dishes and hands, they are often better for the environment.

Basics

Garlic press, cutting boards, vegetable peeler, mixing bowls and measuring spoons, strainer, salad spinner, multi-use grater, rice cooker (though a multi-use electric pressure cooker can do both!).

Optional

Juicer, mortar & pestle, and indoor grill.

APPENDIX E

Simple Swaps for Everyday Life

Our world is so heavily inundated with toxins that there's simply no way to be completely free of them. At work, at school, out traveling and eating at the mercy of restaurants—our detox pathways are constantly at work.

Even if you build a brand new home with conscientious materials, excellent air filtration, green furniture, and only the best products come through the door, you're still contending with outside air, junk coming in on your feet and your clothes, and more.

But we can make simple swaps, one at a time, that eventually add up to make a difference. Here are some low-toxin or toxin-clearing ideas in each category we've covered, to help get you started.

Food

Grow your own food and fall in love with your own, organic garden. If you don't have room for a garden, consider raised beds, patio and container gardens—at least seasonally!

Community gardens are another option and are gaining popularity in neighborhoods and in urban areas.

Grow your own low-light herbs and vegetables indoors from organic and non-GMO seeds to avoid pollutants and pesticides.

Prepare meals in bulk, weekly or monthly, to lessen your need for convenience food.

Water

Ideally, all your water would come from a clean spring. This water would have its mineral content retained, and it wouldn't need to be filtered. Look for a spring near you via www.findaspring.com. Purchase spring water when out to dinner.

Carbon-filtered water is the easiest, next-best option for personal consumption at home.

If you own your own home, consider a whole-home filter to remove pollutants not only from your drinking water, but the water you use to clean your clothes and dishes and in which you bathe and shower.

Advanced methods for water purification include Reverse Osmosis and distillation, but both can deplete your water of minerals and can be cumbersome in the home.

Personal Care Products

Support artisans who make natural, reliable personal care products, including deodorant, shampoo, conditioner, lotion, salves, balms, fragrances, cosmetics, and more. Look for them in local markets, health food stores, and online. Ingredients should be clear, simple, and ideally, things you would not be afraid to consume orally.

Learn to make your own balms using melted coconut oil, shea butter, beeswax, and essential oils.

Use Castile soap on its own or as a base for homemade shampoos and conditioners.

Household Products

In place of chemically-produced, commercial cleaning products, use baking soda, vinegar, and water for basic cleaning and scrubbing.

Make or purchase cleaner sprays with only water, alcohol, and essential oils.

Infuse fragrant herbs or orange peels into vinegar as a cleaner spray.

Use infused-herb or essential-oil based freshening sprays instead of conventional air-fresheners.

For deeper cleans (for example, to target shower mildew and to clean toilets), seek out the purest products with as few chemicals as possible to get the job done. But you'll likely be surprised at how effective natural products can be in cleaning your home.

In-Home Air

A whole-home air exchange system is an option, but pricey and sometimes unattainable—particularly if you live in an apartment.

Remember, your primary goal should not be to filter your air, but rather to recycle your air, exchanging indoor with outdoor air several times per day. In-home filtration is an added bonus.

In the absence of an whole-home air exchange system, there are simple steps you can take:

- Open your windows as often as possible.
- Keep leafy house plants wherever you can.
- Replace carpets with solid-surface floors.
- Air out new furniture before permanently situating it in your home.
- Keep your air return filter and ceiling fan blades clean.
- Minimize electronics, especially in closed spaces.

APPENDIX F

Quick Reference Exercise Guide

Prioritize surges of high-intensity, high-energy movements over prolonged cardio. Work within your existing fitness levels and gradually stretch them over time. Include workouts a few times a week within a lifestyle of movement (walk the stairs instead of the elevator, sit on an exercise ball instead of an office chair or the couch) and flexibility.

Cardiovascular Surge Training

Focus on full body movements that vary in time (duration), tempo (intensity), and type of exercise (see examples below). Experiment with other types of surges (HIIT, tabata), within this basic framework: Aim for 80% Maximum Heart Rate during the sets. Vary intensity by skill level while maintaining consistent rest periods and reps.

To Calculate Your Target Heart Rate (THR):

- Calculate your maximum heart rate (MHR) by subtracting your age from the number 220.
- Your target heart rate (THR) in surge cycles should be 80% of your MHR.
- During rest periods, you can check your heart rate to ensure you are approximating your THR during periods of exertion.

How to Surge Train:

1. Intense movement for 20 seconds
2. Rest for 20 seconds
3. Repeat 3 times
4. Rest for 1–4 minutes, based on exertion and skill
5. Repeat for 5–6 exercises or about 12–15 minutes of exertion

Examples of Surges:

- Sprints
- Uphill walking
- Running in place in the pool
- Swimming laps
- Stationary bike
- Stairmill
- Elliptical
- Any other cardio equipment

Strength Training

The intent of this section is not to give you anatomical guides to every possible exercise. No amount of pictures or instructions in a book can ensure you are exercising safely and properly! When beginning any type of weight training program, work with a coach or a trainer, or at least follow some of the more detailed exercise guides, programs, and demonstrations available on MaxLiving.com.

Whether you are looking to commence a strength training regimen, get back into a routine, or refine yours to incorporate the principles of surge training—which will also be much more effective for your time—use the following as a guide.

Body Balance

Given how much people now sit and use computers, everyone should consider exercising their posterior chain (the back of the body) twice as hard or twice as much as their anterior chain (the front of the body). Because men typically gain weight above the belt while women typically gain weight below the belt, men and women should focus a greater amount of time on these areas, proportionately.

Before determining the types and numbers of exercise sets you'll perform, depending on your goals and time constraints, ensure you've laid out a routine that serves to balance your body.

Upper Body Example

The noted graphics depict just one set of well-rounded upper body exercises, but specific movements for muscle groups should be varied as often as possible. And, as a bonus, full-body functional movements force you to pair up complementary parts of the body, pairing primary and secondary muscles while stabilizing core muscles. Look up more exercises on MaxLiving.com.

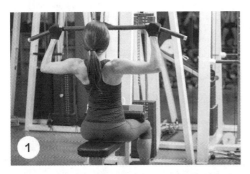

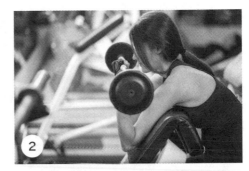

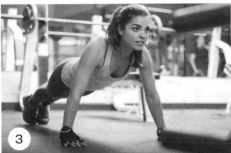

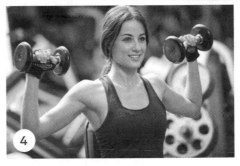

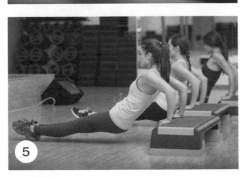

1. Back exercise (posterior chain) using equipment: Lat Pull-Down
2. Bicep exercise using a barbell: Seated Preacher Curl
3. Chest exercise (anterior chain) using bodyweight: Push-Up
4. Shoulder exercise using dumbbells: Overhead Press
5. Tricep exercise using bodyweight: Seated Dips

High-Efficiency Quick Sets

The days of doing "five sets of ten" are long over. Remember: long, drawn out exercises can have a negative impact on the gut and can spike the stress hormone cortisol, which actually promotes fat storage. By surging muscle activity through high-efficiency quick sets, you increase the release of growth hormone and testosterone to promote muscle development without the negative consequences of longer workouts. These also more closely model the body's innate style of exercising—going all out until you hit fatigue before moving on to your next exercise.

Surge Set

Just as you did in cardio surge training, aim for 20 seconds at a time, with 20 second breaks. This type of set can be done with weights or your own bodyweight.

1. Intense muscular exertion for 20 seconds (maintain good form, but go fast).
2. Rest for 20 seconds.
3. Repeat 5 times.

By the time you've done 5-6 sets of 20 seconds, you shouldn't be able to do any more. If this was easy, be sure to increase your weight or number of sets next time.

Drop Set

Incorporate this type of set specifically when you are using weights.

1. Intense muscular exertion for 8-12 repetitions, reaching failure (inability to do more).
2. Rest approximately 10 seconds.
3. Lower the weight 10-20%.
4. Repeat 2-3 times.

On the fourth set, you will have dropped your weight approximately 30%-50% from your first rep. But because your sets are short, with very little break in between them, you should be exhausted after four sets.

Rep Reduction Set

This is an easy set-grouping you can do with weights or with your own bodyweight.

1. Intense muscular exertion for 8–12 repetitions, reaching failure (inability to do more).
2. Rest approximately 10 seconds.
3. Maintaining your weight, reduce the number of repetitions by 2–3.
4. Repeat 3–4 times.

By the fourth or fifth set, you should have dropped down to only one or two repetitions, but with the same amount of weight. If you're working hard enough, you should reach fatigue, and will not be able to do any more.

Flexibility

Stretching may be the most primal form of self-care. For every body part that you work to strengthen, you should also work to stretch. Whole-body stretching should be practiced daily.

As with strength training by body part, one can also break stretches down by muscle group, but full-body motions are most ideal. And, for the same reason your strengthening exercises should emphasize the posterior chain (back of the body) due to modernized postures and routines, you should give your anterior chain extra attention when stretching.

Always, it is best to work with a practitioner to establish a personalized routine based on your body's needs. Keep contrasting muscle groups in mind to ensure you are looking after your entire self—not just where you "feel it."

Upper Body

- **Anterior Chain**
  - Forward Shoulders
  - Pectorals (chest)
  - Biceps
  - Abdominals
- **Posterior Chain**
  - Back Shoulders
  - Latissimus Dorsi (back)
  - Triceps

Lower Body

- **Anterior Chain**
  - Quadriceps (front of thighs)
  - Lower leg (front)
- **Posterior Chain**
  - Buttocks
  - Hamstrings (back of thighs)
  - Calves

APPENDIX G

Meal Planning for Success

Weekly Meal Planning Tips

Map out your meal plan one week in advance.

Do your shopping and meal prep on Saturdays or Sundays, so that your week of eating runs smoothly.

Plan out your meals and shopping list to include ingredients that will be used for multiple meals throughout the week, plus dinners that can be later served as lunch leftovers.

Plan on making simpler meals Monday through Friday, while getting creative on Saturday and Sunday when you have more time. Simple salads, smoothies, chia and hemp puddings, scrambled eggs, yogurt and coconut milk yogurt are great breakfast and lunch staples throughout the week. For dinner, stick with clean protein choices, tons of veggies and great fats.

To avoid food sensitivities—which develop over time—avoid having the same foods every day. Remember that the body was also designed to consume varying foods with the change of the seasons—doing this is also thought to help prevent food sensitivities. When introducing any new foods into your diet, or when reintroducing any foods in the recovery from prior sensitivities, the optimal spacing occurs over four days, so that you can monitor your body's response.

Be sure to include healthy fat, fiber, and protein in every meal.

Avoid repeating core ingredients in your breakfast, lunch, and dinner.

Consume nutrient-dense, full meals to prevent yourself from snacking in between them. Meals loaded with healthy fats and adequate amounts of fiber and protein are primed to keep you full.

You can easily add cold organic chicken, pasture-raised hard boiled eggs, hemp seeds and/or raw nuts to any lunch salad if you need additional protein on workout days (or to stay full.) Great fats that can be added to any salad include: sprouted flax meal, chia seeds, avocado, coconut, and olives.

If you must snack, avoid consuming higher-sugar carbohydrates by themselves, as to not affect insulin levels. On the other hand, raw vegetables are your most ideal carbs; the more you can keep around for snacks—particularly for kids— the better. Liberally consume green beans, raw jicama, bell peppers, cauliflower, cucumber with any snack or on their own, keeping you full and having nearly zero impact on your caloric intake.

Keep your hormones in check by not eating after dinner.

If you choose to fast, aim to have two meals within your day (instead of three) within a six-to-eight hour time frame. When not fasting, follow a regimen of three meals per day and ensure your meals are filling enough to keep you full for four to six hours.

When you do feel the urge to snack, avoid consuming carbohydrates by themselves—and be sure that your craving isn't something that can be resolved with some flat or sparkling water.

The table below shows three unique meals and one unique optional snack for every day of a seven-day week. This is likely more variety than you will need, but enough to serve as a baseline formula for success, while demonstrating that eating the MaxLiving way need not ever be boring.

All meals within the table below are approved on both the MaxLiving Core and Advanced Nutrition Plans.

Sample One Week Meal Plan				
	Breakfast	Lunch	Optional Snack	Dinner
Monday	Coconut Hemp Porridge	Broccoli Cranberry Salad	Baba Ganoush with Veggies	Black Bean Burgers in Maximized Grainless Rolls
Tuesday	Eggs over Spinach with Berries	Garden Salad with Organic Chicken or Hemp Seeds	Almond Power Bar	Advanced Plan "Mac" & Cheese
Wednesday	Chia Seed Pudding	Not Tuna Salad	Granny Smith Apple with Pumpkin Seed Butter	Asian Turkey Lettuce Wraps
Thursday	Grainless Granola with Yogurt and Berries	Sweet & Savory Salad	Apple Flaxseed Muffin	Chicken, Steak or Lentil Walnut Balls with Grilled Veggies
Friday	Mint Chocolate Dream Smoothie	Lime & Walnut Coleslaw	Red Peppers with Tahini	Fish Fry Dinner
Saturday	Coconut Milk & Curry Frittata	Cream of Tomato Soup	Nine-Layer Taco Dip with Veggies	Maximized Shepherd's Pie
Sunday	Maximized Blueberry Pancakes	Grain-Free Cauliflower Tabbouleh	Hummus with Veggies	Herb Butter Salmon & Asparagus

Part Four

Recipes

Breakfast

Maximized Blueberry Pancakes

Asparagus Frittata

Chia Seed Pudding

Zucchini Fritter Cups

Mini Onion Quiches

Grainless Granola

Coconut Milk and Curry Frittata

Coconut Hemp Porridge

Almond Power Bars

 Core Plan   Advanced Plan   Raw **V** Vegan 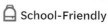 School-Friendly

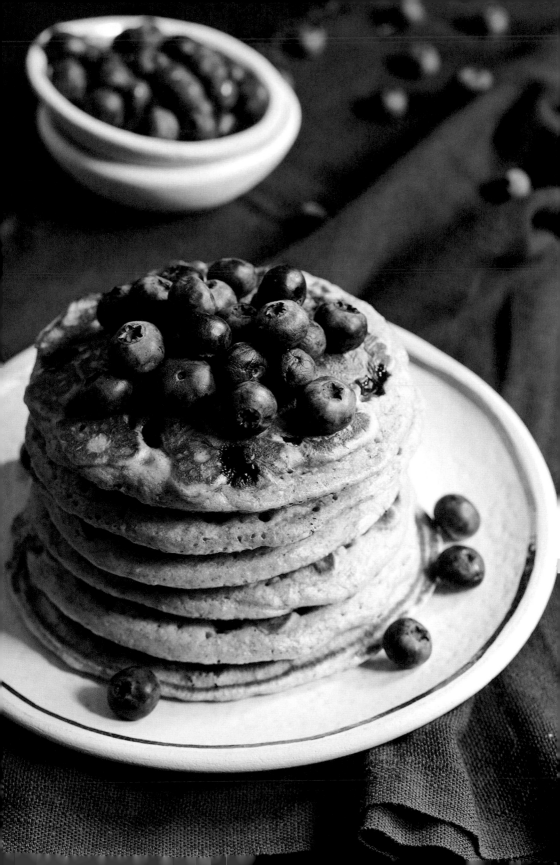

Maximized Blueberry Pancakes

Delicious blueberries mixed in with the light flavor and airy texture of coconut flour will make this recipe your new favorite breakfast or snack! These blueberry pancakes are free from wheat and other grains, and almond flour and coconut flour have a low score on the glycemic index.

1 cup almond flour

1 tablespoon coconut flour, finely ground

1 teaspoon baking powder

Pinch of Himalayan sea salt

3 organic, pasture-raised eggs

¼ cup full fat organic milk

4 drops liquid stevia

Seeds scraped from one vanilla bean

⅓ cup fresh organic blueberries

1 tablespoon coconut oil for greasing

½ cup fresh organic blueberries for topping

SERVES 2

Directions

In a medium bowl, combine the almond flour, coconut flour, salt, and baking powder. Set aside.

Place the eggs, stevia drops, vanilla, and milk in a small bowl and whisk well.

Add egg mixture to dry ingredients, whisk until just combined, do not overmix. Gently stir in the blueberries.

Preheat a large pan over medium heat. Lightly grease the pan with coconut oil.

For each pancake, spoon ¼ cup of the pancake mixture onto pan. Cook until surface of pancakes have some bubbles and sides of the pancake firm up, about 2–3 minutes.

Carefully flip the pancakes with a thin spatula, and cook the underside, for another 45 seconds. Continue with remaining mixture.

Serve the pancakes warm, topped with fresh blueberries.

Asparagus Frittata

Everyone enjoys the beautiful look of asparagus frittata, not to mention the delectable savory taste. Use this tasty dish as the centerpiece at your next brunch.

2 teaspoons olive oil

1 small yellow onion, or two small shallots, thinly sliced

½ teaspoon Himalayan sea salt

1 pound asparagus, tough ends snapped off, spears cut diagonally into 1-inch lengths

4–6 large organic, pasture-raised eggs, lightly beaten

1 cup shredded raw organic gruyere or swiss cheese

SERVES 3–4

Directions

Preheat oven to 450°F.

Gently heat olive oil into a 10-inch ovenproof frying pan over medium-high heat.

Add onions and salt and cook, stirring occasionally, until onions are softened, about 3 minutes.

Add asparagus, reduce heat to medium-low, and cook, covered, until the asparagus are slightly tender, 6–8 minutes.

Pour in eggs and cook until almost set, but still runny on top, about 2 minutes.

Sprinkle cheese over eggs and put in oven to bake uncovered until eggs are set and cheese is melted and browned, about 5–7 minutes. You may want to turn on the broiler during this baking time to better brown the top.

Remove from oven and slide frittata onto a serving plate. Cut into wedges and serve.

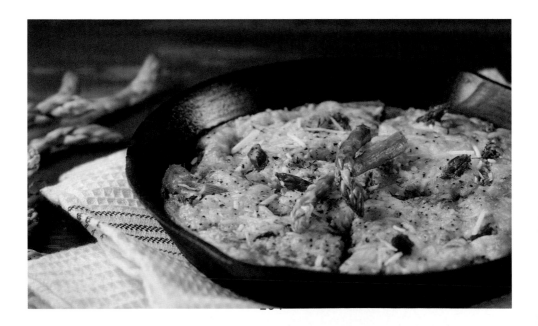

Chia Seed Pudding

  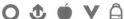

Chia seeds are very versatile. Use them as an egg substitute, sprinkle them into your protein shake, add them into recipes, and fit them into your eating plan however you can. Try this chia seed pudding for a quick and easy breakfast.

1 can coconut milk

¼ cup chia seeds

1 teaspoon organic vanilla

1 teaspoon cinnamon

SERVES 4–6

Directions

Combine all ingredients in a mixing bowl or a blender.

Cover and place in the refrigerator to thicken.

Serve topped with cacao, raw unsweetened coconut flakes, dried fruits, berries, or nuts.

Zucchini Fritter Cups

This flavorful and very easy-to-make recipe is sure to impress guests at your next get-together. These zucchini fritter cups are even a great breakfast option to make ahead of time and have ready for those busy mornings!

2 medium zucchinis, shredded

½ small yellow onion, minced

1 ½ cups almond flour

2 organic, pasture-raised eggs, whisked

2 garlic cloves, minced

1 tablespoon garlic powder

1 teaspoon Himalayan sea salt

Black pepper, to taste

MAKES 7 CUPS

Directions

Preheat oven to 400°F.

Place zucchini and yellow onion in a food processor using the shredding attachment and shred. Place in a couple paper towels and squeeze out all the excess liquid. You may have to replace the paper towels a few times!

Place zucchini and onion in a bowl, mix well with almond flour, egg, garlic cloves, garlic powder, salt and pepper.

Scoop out the mixture and place into 7 muffin cups. Either use silicone muffin liners or be sure to heavily grease each muffin tin to keep it from sticking.

Bake for 25–30 minutes.

Let cool before removing from muffin tin.

Mini Onion Quiches

These mini quiches are great to freeze for a quick on-the-go breakfast later. We substituted a typical crust with shredded coconut.

¾ cup shredded coconut

4 tablespoons butter, melted

1 cup chopped green onions with tops

2 tablespoons butter

2 organic, pasture-raised eggs

1 cup organic whole milk

½ teaspoon Himalayan sea salt

¼ teaspoon pepper

1 cup swiss cheese, grated

Directions

Preheat oven to 300°F. Combine coconut and melted butter. Divide coconut among mini muffin tins. Sauté onion for 10 minutes in 2 tablespoons of butter. Cool onions and divide evenly over coconut crust. Beat eggs, add milk, salt, pepper, and swiss cheese. Pour by spoonfuls on top of onions in the tins. Do not fill to the top as they will run over. Bake until set, about 15–20 minutes. Do not overbake.

MAKES 10–12 QUICHES

Grainless Granola

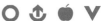

This recipe is a great healthy option for those who miss their morning cereal.

¼ cup whole flaxseeds

¼ cup raw sunflower seeds

¼ cup raw organic almonds or walnuts

¼ cup raw dehydrated coconut flakes, unsweetened

½ can chilled coconut milk

¼ teaspoon cinnamon

SERVES 4

Directions

In a dry blender or food processor, pour flaxseeds, sunflower seeds, almonds, and coconut flakes through opening in top cover. Replace removable cap and continue processing until ingredients are reduced to a chunky, grain-like consistency, about 1 minute. Stop motor, scrape down to loosen mixture in bottom of blender or work bowl, if necessary. Add cinnamon and process a few more bursts until blended. Scoop out 1/2 cup mixture per serving. Pour roughly equal amounts of coconut milk or other milk per serving over cereal and enjoy.

TIP This granola can be enjoyed cold or add coconut milk, let stand a few minutes & warm slightly on stovetop for a hot cereal. Flaxseeds will thicken mixture as it sits.

Coconut Milk and Curry Frittata

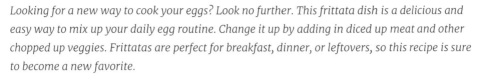

Looking for a new way to cook your eggs? Look no further. This frittata dish is a delicious and easy way to mix up your daily egg routine. Change it up by adding in diced up meat and other chopped up veggies. Frittatas are perfect for breakfast, dinner, or leftovers, so this recipe is sure to become a new favorite.

7 organic, pasture-raised eggs

½ red onion, finely diced

2 cups fresh spinach, chopped

¼ cup coconut milk

2 tablespoons tomato paste

1 tablespoon curry powder

1 tablespoon coconut oil

Himalayan sea salt, to taste

SERVES 6

Directions

Heat the coconut oil in a medium sized skillet, add the onions, and cook until the onions begin to caramelize.

While the onions are cooking, whisk together the eggs, coconut milk, tomato paste, curry powder, and salt.

Add the spinach to the onions and oil and cook until the spinach is wilted.

Evenly spread the onion and spinach mixture over the bottom of the skillet and pour in the egg mixture.

Cover and cook over medium low heat for 4 minutes.

Transfer the frittata to the oven and cook under the broiler, uncovered, for another 2–3 minutes or until the frittata is cooked all the way through.

Cut into wedges and serve.

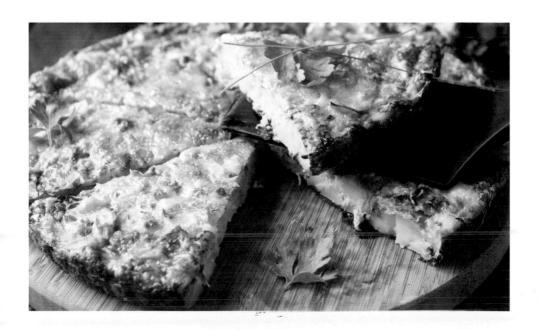

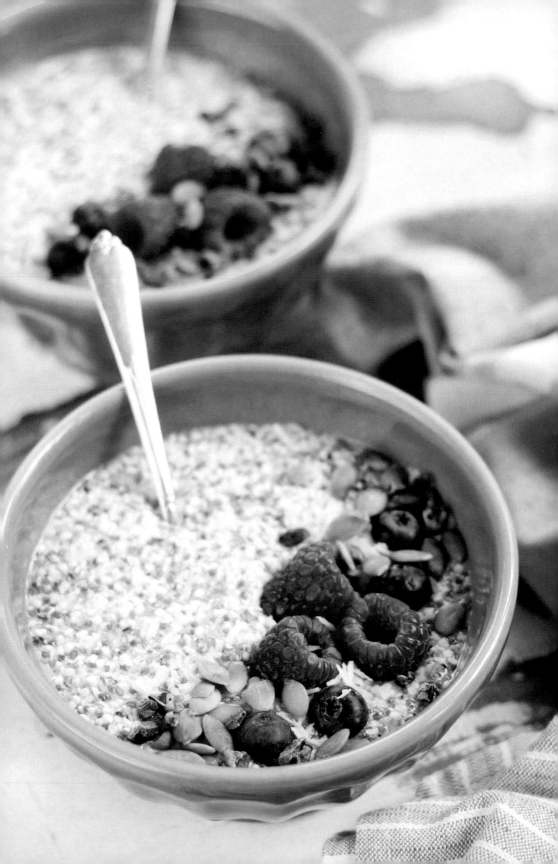

Coconut Hemp Porridge

Porridge is one of the most filling breakfasts and is a great way to start your busy mornings. Go grain-free with this coconut hemp porridge recipe. This scrumptious meal will keep you full and can also be served for lunch or as a snack.

1 cup nut milk (e.g. coconut milk)

½ cup raw, shelled hemp seeds

¼ cup shredded coconut, unsweetened

1 tablespoon chia seeds

1 tablespoon flaxseed meal

4–6 drops stevia, to taste

1 teaspoon pure vanilla extract

½ teaspoon cinnamon

Pinch of Himalayan sea salt

SERVES 2–4

Directions

Combine all ingredients (except toppings) in a small saucepan. Stir well and bring to a boil over medium heat.

Keep stirring and reduce heat to medium-low. Allow porridge to simmer until it thickens, about 2–4 minutes.

Pour into serving bowls, add toppings of your choice, and serve immediately.

Optional toppings

Fresh berries, pumpkin seeds, chopped raw nuts

TIP If you are taking this to work, make it the evening before.

Almond Power Bars

These protein bars can be enjoyed with or without the chocolate topping. They make a wonderful lunchbox treat, but you do need to ensure that they stay cold. Take an ice pack with you to make sure these delicious bars keep throughout the day.

2 cups raw almonds

½ cup flaxseed meal

½ cup unsweetened shredded coconut

2 scoops of organic, grass-fed whey protein in the flavor of your choice

½ cup raw almond butter

½ teaspoon Himalayan sea salt

½ cup coconut oil

⅛ teaspoon of stevia, (equivalent to approximately ½ cup of sugar). Taste and adjust to your liking.

1 tablespoon pure vanilla extract (sugar-free – check the label)

Raw nuts and raw nut butters such as macadamia (optional)

MAKES 20–24 SQUARES

Directions

Place almonds, flaxseed meal, shredded coconut, organic, grass-fed whey protein, almond butter, and salt in a food processor. Add in raw nuts and raw nut butters as desired.

Pulse briefly, about 10 seconds.

In a small saucepan, melt coconut oil over very low heat. Remove coconut oil from stove; stir stevia and vanilla into oil.

Add coconut oil mixture to food processor and pulse until ingredients form a coarse paste.

Press mixture into an 8 × 8 inch glass baking dish (parchment paper liner helps you remove the bars from the dish).

Chill in refrigerator for 1 hour, until mixture hardens.

Optional topping

8 squares unsweetened chocolate, melted and sweetened to taste with stevia and cinnamon

In a double boiler, melt chocolate. Stir in stevia and cinnamon.

Spread melted chocolate over bars; return to refrigerator for 30 minutes until chocolate hardens.

Remove from refrigerator, cut into bars, and serve.

Smoothies & Beverages

Simple Smoothie

Avocado Green Smoothie

Amaretto Cappuccino Smoothie

Raspberry Explosion

Pumpkin Spice Smoothie

Apple-Almond Smoothie

Mint Chocolate Dream

Ginger Switchel

Apple Cinnamon Elixir

Sugar-free Lemonade

Cinnamon Citrus Cider

Sparkling Raspberry Lemonade

Coconut Milk Hot Cocoa

 Core Plan   Advanced Plan   Raw   V Vegan   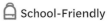 School-Friendly

Simple Smoothie

Smoothies are the best way to start your day! You can add in a ton of great ingredients to make a different smoothie every day. Here's a basic smoothie recipe and a list of other ingredients you can add for flavor and more good healthy fats.

1 scoop vanilla organic, grass-fed whey protein powder

½ can unsweetened full-fat coconut milk

½ cup filtered water

½ cup frozen berries (blackberries, blueberries, and raspberries)

Directions

Combine in blender coconut milk, filtered water, and berries. Blend on high until well blended.

Add vanilla protein powder and blend for 10 seconds.

Add optional ingredients and blend.

Serve immediately.

SERVES 1

Optional ingredients

1 cup raw yogurt

½ avocado

1 handful of spinach

¼ cup flaxseed

2 organic, pasture-raised eggs

1 tablespoon coconut oil or flaxseed oil

1 tablespoon nut butter

Fresh grated ginger

Raw cacao powder or cocoa powder

Almond butter

Ground cinnamon, nutmeg, or allspice

Avocado Green Smoothie

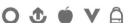

Try this maximized version of your favorite green shake!
Naturally green and ultra-creamy, this shake will surely become a year-round favorite.

1 organic avocado

1 ½ cups ice

1 cup organic spinach

A few drops of peppermint oil/extract

Stevia to taste

Cacao nibs (optional)

Directions

Add all ingredients to blender and mix until smooth.

Additional liquid such as water or almond milk may be required to allow for easier blending.

Serve chilled in a tall glass with or without ice.

SERVES 1

Amaretto Cappuccino Smoothie

If you were wondering if there was a way to maximize an iced cappuccino, here it is! This smoothie is the perfect pick-me-up on a hot summer's day — or anytime.

¾ cup unsweetened almond milk

¼ cup coconut milk

1 scoop chocolate organic, grass-fed whey protein

1 teaspoon instant espresso powder

1 tablespoon spoonable stevia, or equivalent, or to taste

1 teaspoon raw almond butter

4 strong coffee "ice cubes" — see directions

SERVES 1

Directions

Ahead of time, prepare an ice cube tray with strong coffee and freeze ahead.

Use approximately 1 ¼ cups of water to 3 generous teaspoons of instant espresso powder, and mix the coffee in a drinking glass before pouring it into the ice cube tray.

Adjust the strength of the coffee to your taste. Once frozen, keep the coffee ice cubes in a resealable plastic bag in the freezer.

Place all ingredients in a blender and blend until smooth.

TIP Don't consume after 3:00 p.m.

Raspberry Explosion

For the raspberry lover, try out this delicious fruity breakfast smoothie.

1–2 scoops berry flavored organic, grass-fed whey protein powder

3 tablespoons full fat organic yogurt

1/4 – 1/2 cup frozen or fresh berries

Water to desired consistency

1/2 – 1 teaspoon spoonable stevia

1 teaspoon greens powder (optional)

1 teaspoon hemp seed oil (optional)

Directions

Mix everything together in a blender or Vitamix®. Add water or ice and blend to desired consistency.

SERVES 1

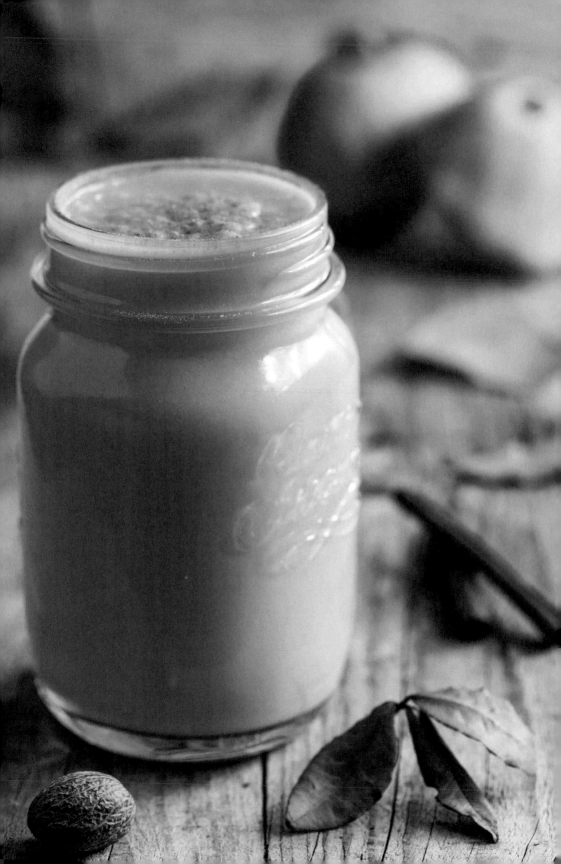

◀ Pumpkin Spice Smoothie

Fuel your body with this delicious fall-inspired protein shake. Just toss these few simple ingredients into your blender and you'll have a healthy treat for breakfast or after a workout!

1 cup coconut milk

½ cup pumpkin puree

½ teaspoon cinnamon

½ teaspoon nutmeg

1 ½ scoops organic, grass-fed whey protein

A little sprinkle of nutmeg for topping

Directions

Combine all ingredients in a high-speed blender and blend until desired texture.

SERVES 1–2

> **TIP** You can also place the smoothie mixture in an ice cream maker for pumpkin spice ice cream.

Apple-Almond Smoothie

Enjoy this satisfying apple-almond breakfast smoothie. Add organic, grass-fed whey or hemp protein for extra protein.

Handful of greens (swiss chard, spinach, kale)

¼ – ½ cup coconut milk

1 banana, sliced

Spoonful almond butter

1 apple, peeled

Directions

Put everything in the blender and blend for 30–45 seconds. Add water or ice to reach desired consistency.

SERVES 1

Mint Chocolate Dream

Try out this breakfast smoothie that really tastes like a dessert!

1–2 scoops chocolate organic, grass-fed whey protein powder

¼ – ½ can coconut milk

1 tablespoon mint-flavored greens powder

1 teaspoon organic cocoa

½ – 1 teaspoon spoonable stevia

1 tablespoon hemp seed oil (optional)

1 teaspoon almond butter (optional)

Directions

Mix everything together in a blender or Vitamix®. Add water or ice and blend to desired consistency.

SERVES 1

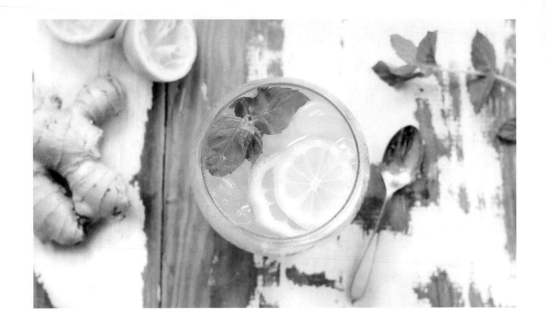

Ginger Switchel

Switchel originated in the Caribbean and has been a popular summer drink for centuries. Farmers call it "Haymaker's Punch" as it is popular at harvest time. Use stevia instead of traditional honey to keep it maximized.

2 tablespoons apple cider vinegar

12 drops of liquid stevia

¼ teaspoon ground ginger or 1 teaspoon grated fresh ginger

1 cup water

½ organic lemon

SERVES 1–2

Directions

Combine all ingredients in a jar or a glass.

Cover and refrigerate at least 2 hours and up to a day.

Shake or stir before serving.

Taste and adjust stevia amount, if desired.

If using fresh ginger, strain through a fine sieve or cheesecloth.

Pour over ice or mix with soda water, if desired.

Apple Cinnamon Elixir

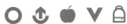

This recipe is a simple way to get your fix of these awesome nutrients for hectic mornings. Sip this drink steaming as a morning or as bedtime cool down drink. If you prefer, sweeten it with stevia or raw honey.

1–2 tablespoons organic apple cider vinegar

1 tablespoon lemon juice

1 teaspoon cinnamon

2 cups boiling water

Liquid stevia, raw organic honey, or unrefined maple syrup (optional — Core Plan only)

Directions

Stir ingredients together and drink in the morning or before bedtime.

Serve warm or cool.

SERVES 1–2

Sugar-free Lemonade

This sugar-free recipe is quick and easy-to-make with all the healthy benefits of lemons. Enjoy this healthier, natural twist on a classic favorite served alongside a grilled meal.

1 cup pure lemon juice

2 cups water

1 cup ice

Stevia and mint leaves, to taste

Directions

Stir and garnish with a slice of lemon.

SERVES 1–2

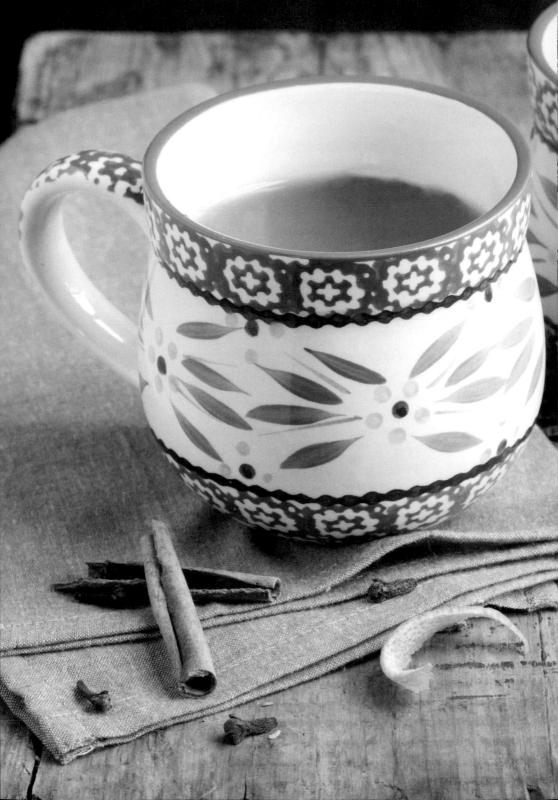

Cinnamon Citrus Cider

Nothing says fall like a cup of hot apple cider on a chilly autumn or winter day!
This recipe provides you with a friendly version of your favorite fall comfort beverage.
Keep it warm in a crock pot to serve at your holiday get-together or store in the fridge.

5 cups organic apple cider

1 cinnamon stick

2 whole cloves

1 (½ inch thick) orange
slice with peel

1 (½ inch thick) lemon
slice with peel

¼ teaspoon
ground nutmeg

Cinnamon sticks and/
or thinly sliced apples
for garnish (optional)

Directions

Combine cider, cinnamon stick, cloves, orange slice, lemon slice, and nutmeg in a medium saucepan. Bring to a boil.

Cover, reduce heat, and simmer 20 minutes.

Strain cider mixture through a sieve into a bowl and discard solids.

Garnish each serving with 1 cinnamon stick and a thin slice of apple, if desired.

SERVES 4–6

Sparkling Raspberry Lemonade ○ ⚓ V 🅰

Perfect for summertime — or any time of the year — this lemonade is an easy and delicious party drink that will be a hit with both children and adults. This refreshing, flavorful mix is sweetened with xylitol so you can relax and enjoy your favorite summer drink worry-free!

1 12-ounce package frozen unsweetened raspberries (about 3 cups)

1 cup xylitol

½ cup water

1 ½ tablespoons grated lemon peel

1 cup fresh lemon juice

1 1-liter bottle chilled sparkling water or club soda

Ice cubes

Fresh raspberries (optional)

Lemon slices

SERVES 6

Directions

Combine frozen raspberries, xylitol, and ½ cup water in medium saucepan.

Stir over medium heat until xylitol dissolves and berries thaws and boil 3 minutes.

Strain raspberry mixture into bowl, pressing on solids to extract as much liquid as possible. Discard solids in strainer.

Mix lemon peel into raspberry syrup in bowl. Chill until cold.

Stir raspberry syrup, lemon juice, and sparkling water in large pitcher to blend.

Fill 6 glasses with ice cubes. Pour raspberry lemonade into glasses.

Add fresh raspberries to each glass, if desired. Garnish with lemon slices and serve.

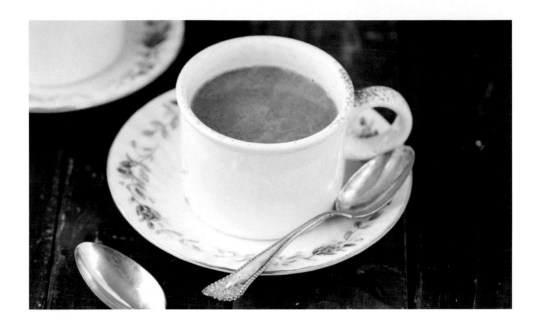

Coconut Milk Hot Cocoa

Nothing says cozy like a delicious cup of hot cocoa and a warm blanket on a cold winter's night. Enjoy the comfort of hot chocolate with this healthy alternative. Serve it in a glass or travel mug for your on-the-go activities. It's sure to boost your morning!

⅓ cup full fat unsweetened coconut milk

⅔ cup boiling water

1 tablespoon unsweetened cocoa powder

1 teaspoon vanilla

15 drops liquid stevia

SERVES 1–2

Directions

Combine and stir coconut milk, boiling water, unsweetened cocoa powder, and vanilla together.

Serve with whipped cream made of organic heavy cream, and sprinkle with cacao nibs, if desired.

Optional toppings

1–2 drops peppermint oil, whipped cream, cacao nibs

TIP For a creamier hot chocolate, you can use more coconut milk and less water.

Soups

Butternut Squash and Leek Soup

Homemade Chicken Broth

Chilled Cream of Tomato Soup

Red Lentil Tomato Kale Soup

Italian Spinach Soup

Cream of Cauliflower Soup

Chicken Sausage Soup

 Core Plan 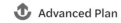 Advanced Plan Raw Vegan 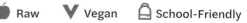 School-Friendly

Butternut Squash and Leek Soup

Even if you think you don't like squash, this is a delicious soup.
It's very creamy without the use of milk or cream.

1 head of garlic

2 cups water

4 teaspoons olive oil

2 cups organic
chicken broth

6 large leeks, thinly sliced

½ teaspoon
Himalayan sea salt

4 cups butternut
squash (1 squash)

½ teaspoon ground
black pepper

SERVES 4–6

Directions

Preheat oven to 350°F.

Cut squash in half and brush with some olive oil.
Place cut side down on a baking dish and bake for about
30–40 minutes or until squash is soft. Scoop out squash
and set aside.

Remove the white papery skin from garlic head but do
not peel or separate the cloves. Wrap head in foil. Bake
at 350°F for 1 hour; cool 10 minutes. Separate cloves;
squeeze to extract garlic pulp. Discard skins.

Heat oil in a large saucepan over medium-high heat.
Add leek; sauté 5 minutes or until tender.

Stir in garlic, squash, water, broth, salt, and pepper;
bring to a boil. Reduce heat and simmer until well mixed.
Place half the squash mixture in a blender (if the mixture
is still hot you may need to remove the centerpiece of
the blender lid to let steam escape — if so, cover with
a towel instead). Blend until smooth. Repeat procedure
with remaining squash mixture. Do not overcrowd your
blender with hot foods!

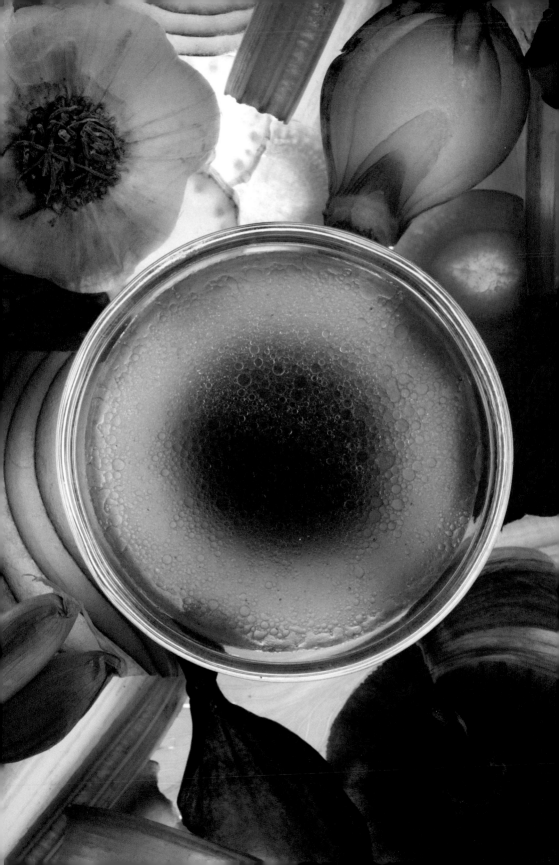

Homemade Chicken Broth

It's difficult to find chicken broth that doesn't contain additives. Fortunately, homemade chicken broth is not difficult to make, and it is well worth the time and easy effort. Once you make a big batch of this golden, hearty broth, you can also freeze it — will be the basis for so many beautiful soups all year long.

2 organic, pasture-raised chicken carcasses

2 small carrots, peeled and trimmed

2 small onions, peeled, trimmed, and quartered

2 small celery stalks, trimmed

3 peeled garlic cloves, smashed

Stems from 1 bunch parsley (optional)

3–4 green leek leaves, sliced (optional)

1 sprig fresh thyme

1 bay leaf

4 quarts water

Directions

In a stockpot, place the chicken bones, then add all of the remaining ingredients, except the water.

Add water to cover by 2 inches, bring to a boil, and reduce the heat. Simmer uncovered for 2 to 3 hours, skimming as necessary.

Strain through a fine-mesh strainer into a clean bowl and cool.

Refrigerate, covered, for up to 3 days, discarding the hardened layer of fat before using or freezing.

SERVES 2–4

Chilled Cream of Tomato Soup

Cold soups are great for hot summer days or for packing in a portable lunch. This raw food soup is full of valuable nutrients.

3 ripe tomatoes, seeded and chopped (about 1 ½ cups)

¼ teaspoon Himalayan sea salt

¼ cup water

½ ripe avocado, chopped

½ teaspoon crushed garlic (1 clove)

1 tablespoons extra virgin olive oil

¼ teaspoon onion powder

2 teaspoon minced fresh dill weed or basil

Directions

Place the tomatoes, water, garlic, onion powder, and salt in a blender and process until smooth. Add avocado and olive oil and blend again until smooth. Add the dill weed and blend briefly, just to mix.

Serve immediately or chill in refrigerator.

SERVES 2–4

Red Lentil Tomato Kale Soup

This hearty, vegan soup is an ideal lunch for colder days, and works as a great side dish for any meal. It's filling, well-balanced, and delicious!

1 teaspoon coconut oil

2 large garlic cloves, minced

1 onion, diced

3 celery stalks, diced

1 teaspoon ground cumin

2 teaspoon chili powder

14 oz canned tomatoes, diced

5–6 cups vegetable broth (more if desired)

1 cup red lentils, rinsed and drained

2 handfuls of torn kale or spinach

Himalayan sea salt and pepper, to taste

Directions

In a large pot, sauté the onion and garlic in oil for about 5–6 minutes over medium heat.

Add in the celery and sauté for a few minutes more.

Stir in the cumin and chili powder.

Stir in the can of tomatoes (including the juice), broth, and lentils. Bring to a boil, reduce heat, and then simmer, uncovered, for about 20–25 minutes, until lentils are tender and fluffy.

Stir in kale or spinach and season to taste, adding more spices if you wish.

SERVES 2

Italian Spinach Soup

Also called Italian Wedding Soup, this is a great dish to enjoy all year round.

Meatballs

1 organic, pasture-raised egg

½ cup organic parmesan cheese

1 small onion

1 teaspoon sea salt

½ teaspoon ground black pepper

1 teaspoon garlic powder

2 pounds organic ground turkey

2 tablespoons coconut oil

Soup

1 quart organic chicken broth

1 cup spinach, chopped

1 teaspoon onion powder

1 tablespoon chopped parsley

1 teaspoon Himalayan sea salt

½ teaspoon ground black pepper

½ teaspoon garlic powder

Directions

Meatballs

In a bowl, combine all meatball ingredients. Shape into 1 inch balls. Fry in coconut oil until done. Set aside.

Soup

Mix all soup ingredients in a saucepan and bring to a boil. When spinach is wilted, add the meatballs and serve.

SERVES 4

TIP The meatballs do not contain breadcrumbs so they are a little more fragile. Fry them with care or bake in the oven.

TIP   If you want to use this soup over a few days, leave the spinach out until you are ready to reheat it then add it into the broth as it heats.

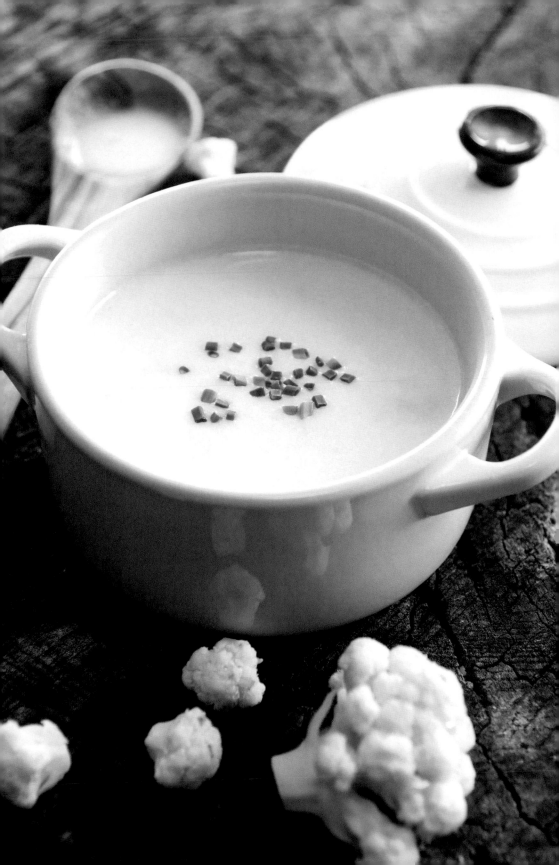

Cream of Cauliflower Soup

Most white foods are typically on the unhealthy list but cauliflower is the exception. Even kids will love this creamy cauliflower soup.

2 cups cauliflower, chopped

1 can coconut milk

½ cup celery, chopped

½ cup onion, chopped

1 teaspoon Himalayan sea salt

⅛ teaspoon ground black pepper

¼ teaspoon curry powder

2 tablespoons organic butter

2 tablespoons coconut flour

1 cup water

Directions

Simmer cauliflower, celery, and onion together in water for 20 minutes or until very tender. Drain and add 1 cup of water.

Purée, a little at a time, in a blender at low speed. Do not overcrowd the blender with hot foods.

Heat butter in a saucepan over medium heat; mix in flour and cook until blended, stirring frequently.

Add coconut milk slowly and stir until smooth.

Mix in purée, salt, pepper, and curry powder, stirring occasionally until hot, but do not boil.

SERVES 4–6

Chicken Sausage Soup

Enjoy this hearty chicken sausage soup. Make sure the chicken or turkey sausage you choose doesn't contain additives like nitrites or pork casings. Read your labels or ask at the meat counter.

1 quart organic chicken broth

1 quart water

6–8 organic chicken or turkey sausage links

3 cloves garlic, sliced

1 medium onion, chopped

2–3 heads escarole or spinach

1 can cannellini beans (white beans), drained

Fresh parsley

Lemon zest

Directions

Brown the onion and garlic in a small amount of olive oil in a medium sized stock pot.

Add chicken stock and water along with salt to taste. Bring to a boil and simmer.

Brown chicken sausages in a separate frying pan and cut into chunks. Set aside.

Add chopped escarole or spinach and cannellini beans to the stock mixture. Let simmer for 5–10 minutes.

Add the sausage right before serving. Top with fresh parsley and lemon zest.

SERVES 4–6

Salads & Slaws

Not Tuna Salad

Lime and Walnut Coleslaw

Grain-Free Cauliflower Tabbouleh

Sweet & Savory Salad

Broccoli Cranberry Salad

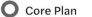 Core Plan   Advanced Plan   Raw **V** Vegan 🎒 School-Friendly

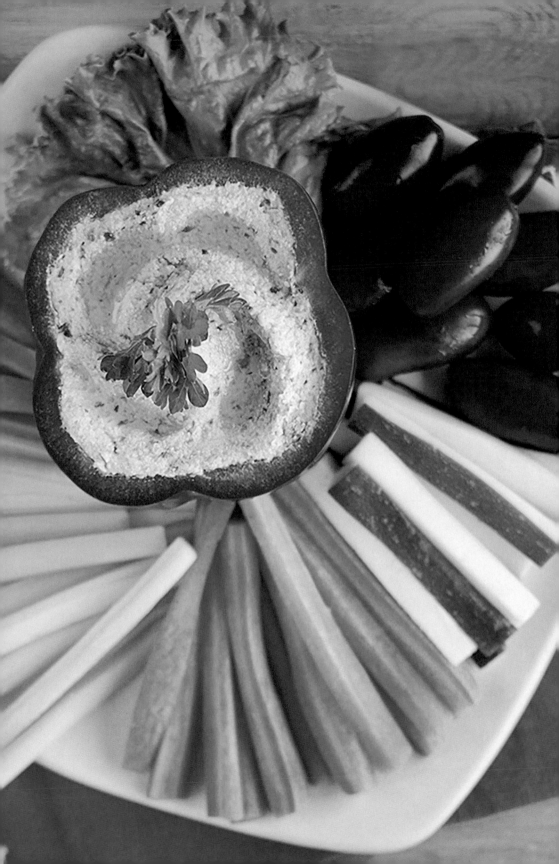

Not Tuna Salad

Looking for something new and delicious to bring for lunch? Take along this great raw, meat-free alternative to tuna salad. Chickpeas are a great source of fiber and protein, especially if you do not eat meat, and sunflower seeds and olive oil will give you your dose of healthy fats. This fresh and tasty Not Tuna Salad recipe works well as a dip with celery or bell peppers, or as filler to your lettuce wrap.

1 cup sunflower seeds, soaked 8–12 hours

1 cup almonds, soaked 8–12 hours

½ cup lemon juice

¼ cup minced celery

2 teaspoons kelp powder

¼ cup minced red onion

¼ cup minced parsley

2 tablespoons minced fresh dill

1 teaspoon Himalayan sea salt

¼ cup olive oil

1 can (1 cup) chickpeas

Directions

Process the almonds, sunflower seeds, sea salt, and lemon juice in a food processor until mixture sticks together in a ball.

You may need to stop the machine and scrape down the walls with a spatula.

Add the remaining ingredients and hand mix.

Optional
Serve in lettuce wraps, endive leaves, or red bell pepper halves.

SERVES 6–8

Lime and Walnut Coleslaw

This coleslaw is sure to be a family favorite. Leave out the jalapeño if you like it milder.

1 ½ cups raw walnut pieces

½ of a medium-large cabbage

1 basket of tiny cherry tomatoes, washed and quartered (optional)

¾ cup cilantro or parsley, chopped

1 small jalapeño pepper, seeded and finely diced (optional)

¼ cup freshly squeezed lime juice

2 tablespoons olive oil

¼ teaspoon Himalayan sea salt

SERVES 6

Directions

Cut the cabbage into two quarters and cut out the core. Using a knife, shred each quarter into thin slices. Ensure they are thin and bite-sized. If any pieces look like they might be too long, cut them in half.

Combine the cabbage, walnuts, tomatoes, jalapeño (optional), and cilantro or parsley in a bowl.

In a separate bowl, combine the lime juice, olive oil, salt. Add to the cabbage mixture and gently stir.

Grain-Free Cauliflower Tabbouleh

Try out this wheat-free and entirely grain-free way to make tabbouleh! Enjoy all the spices and flavors of this mediterranean side dish – it's the perfect appetizer for entertaining. Serve as a salad or even dip for big pieces of vegetables. Not only is it delicious, this dish is very supportive of the detox systems of the body, as it's made with ingredients like parsley, lemon, cilantro, and other raw veggies.

½ large cauliflower, leaves removed

1 ½ cups cherry tomatoes, sliced

½ cup fresh parsley, minced

¾ cups finely chopped celery

⅓ cup cilantro, minced

2 green onions, thinly sliced

2 tablespoons hulled hemp seeds

Himalayan sea salt and pepper, to taste

Juice of 1 whole lemon

Directions

Grate cauliflower on a cheese grater.

Mix all ingredients in a bowl.

Top with juice of a whole lemon and salt and pepper, to taste.

SERVES 2

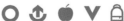

Sweet & Savory Salad

Who doesn't love a sweet and savory combination? This delicious salad gives you the best of both worlds. Serve with organic roasted turkey or wild caught smoked salmon to satisfy meat lovers.

Salad

6 cups organic mixed greens

2 cups organic spinach

1 can (about 2 cups) chickpeas

1–2 granny smith apples

1 cup walnuts, whole or coarsely chopped

4 handfuls blackberries (for garnish)

½ cup organic gorgonzola cheese (optional)

1 avocado, sliced (optional)

Dressing

1 tablespoon grapeseed oil or coconut oil

1 tablespoon grated onion or shallots

1 small clove garlic, minced or pressed

1 pint blackberries

½ cup apple cider vinegar

2 tablespoons balsamic vinegar

½ teaspoon spoonable stevia

½ teaspoon Himalayan sea salt

¼ teaspoon ground black pepper

½ cup olive oil

Directions

In a non-toxic (non-teflon) skillet, make the dressing by heating the grapeseed or coconut oil over medium-high heat. Add the onions (or shallots) and garlic, then cook for about a minute.

Add the blackberries and let break down (about 1–2 min). Pour in both vinegars and stir to combine.

Transfer mixture to a blender or food processor and add the stevia, salt, and pepper.

Blend until smooth and add the olive oil slowly with blender or food processor. If you want to remove all the seeds, strain through a mesh strainer.

Place the greens on a plate. Add remaining ingredients as desired and drizzle with dressing.

For a nice presentation, place apples, blackberries, walnuts, and turkey or salmon (optional) in sections around the edges of the greens.

SERVES 2–4

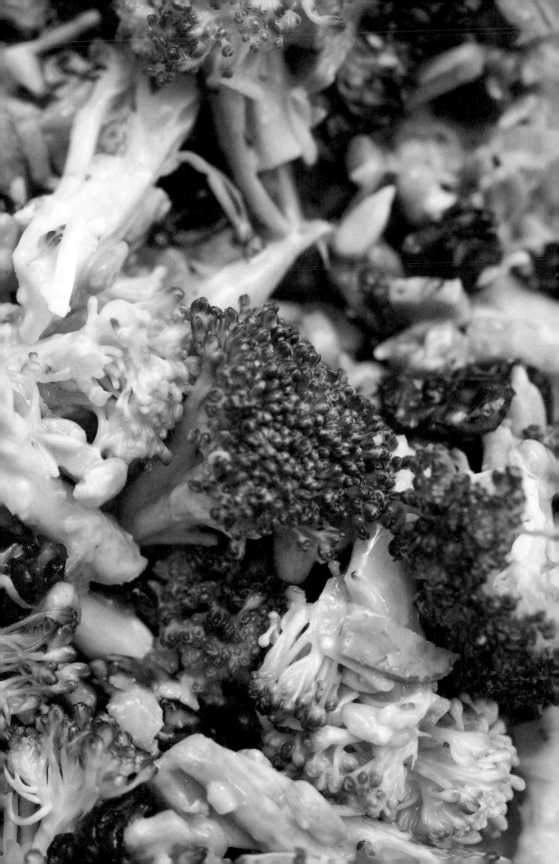

Broccoli Cranberry Salad

Fresh broccoli tossed with cranberries, seeds, turkey bacon, and drizzled with a deliciously creamy dressing makes this salad perfect for BBQs and potlucks. This delectable salad pairs well as a side dish for old fashioned BBQ chicken.

Salad

5 cups raw broccoli florets, chopped

½ cup red onion, chopped

½ cup organic shredded cheese (optional)

1 cup organic turkey bacon, cooked and crumbled

1 cup raw sunflower seeds

1 cup dried cranberries

Dressing

¾ cup organic mayonnaise

Stevia or xylitol to taste

2 tablespoons red wine vinegar

¼ teaspoon red pepper flakes

Directions

Combine all salad ingredients in a large mixing bowl; mix well.

Combine dressing ingredients in a small mixing bowl. Mix until thoroughly combined using a fork or wire whisk.

Add dressing to salad and mix well.

Refrigerate 1 hour.

SERVES 2–4

237

Breads & Baked Goods

Apple Flaxseed Muffins

Savory Raw Flax Crackers

Grain-free Vegan Herb Crackers

Almond Cookies

Almond Flour Flax Meal Pizza Dough

Garlic Parmesan Flaxseed Crackers

Blueberry Muffins

Maximized Grainless Rolls

Cheesy Garlic Coconut Flour Bread

Carrot Cake Muffins

Cranberry Nut Bread

Dark Rye Bread

Chocolate Zucchini Bread

Flax Meal Bread

 Core Plan   Advanced Plan   Raw   **V** Vegan   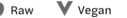 School-Friendly

Apple Flaxseed Muffins

Muffins may seem like cupcakes in disguise, except they are much healthier when maximized like this apple flaxseed muffins recipe. Store them in your freezer so you can pull out one muffin at a time for a delicious snack.

Muffins

1 cup flaxseed meal

2 cups almond meal (can chop raw almonds in food processor)

2 teaspoons aluminum-free baking powder

1 tablespoon cinnamon

¼ teaspoon nutmeg and/or cloves

¼ teaspoon Himalayan sea salt

¼ teaspoon powdered stevia

1 cup xylitol

4–6 large organic, pasture-raised eggs, beaten

½ cup coconut oil

½ cup full-fat organic yogurt

½ cup unsweetened almond milk

2 teaspoons pure vanilla (sugar-free – check the ingredients)

2 medium organic apples, chopped fine

½ cup chopped pecans or walnuts (optional)

½ cup currants (optional on Core Plan only)

Topping

½ cup xylitol

½ teaspoon cinnamon

Directions

Preheat oven to 350°F. Prepare a muffin tin with silicone baking cups or paper liners.

In a food processor, pulse together flaxseed meal, raw almonds, baking powder, cinnamon, nutmeg, salt, stevia, and xylitol.

In a small saucepan, melt coconut oil.

In a separate bowl, mix coconut oil, eggs, almond milk, yogurt, vanilla, apple, nuts, and currants.

Add the wet ingredients to the dry and combine thoroughly. Add additional water or almond milk if too thick.

Let batter stand 10 minutes.

Separate batter into the muffin pan.

Sprinkle on topping.

Bake for approximately 18–20 minutes, or until a toothpick comes out clean.

MAKES 12 MUFFINS

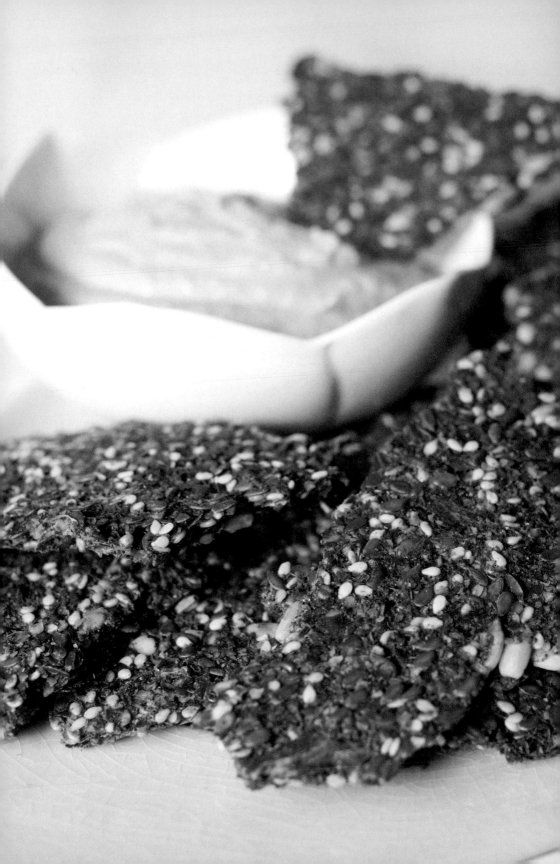

Savory Raw Flax Crackers

High in fiber, nutritious, crunchy, and totally dip-worthy, these crackers are great on their own or paired with hummus or guacamole. The three colors of the seeds add to the appeal, and combination of spices makes these treats deliciously flavorful and impossible to pass up. You will never want to buy boxed crackers again!

1 cup unhulled sesame seeds (to soak – can also use ½ white seeds and ½ black sesame seeds)

2 cups ground brown flaxseeds

1 cup whole brown flaxseeds

1 cup sunflower (or golden flaxseeds), not ground

2 tablespoons cumin (whole, not ground)

1 teaspoon curry powder

1 teaspoon Himalayan sea salt

1 ½ cups water

1 lemon (include peel if lemon is organic)

4 stalks celery

1 large onion

2 large handfuls of your choice of greens (example: kale/spinach)

1 packed cup parsley

1 cup purple carrots (optional)

MAKES FOUR 12×12" SHEETS

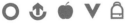

Directions

Soak sesame seeds while preparing other ingredients.

Place flaxseeds, cumin, curry, and salt in a large bowl and stir.

Blend the remaining ingredients except sesame seeds and carrots, then stir into the mixture in the bowl.

Drain and rinse the soaked sesame seeds, then stir into the dough.

Stir in the grated carrots (optional).

Allow to sit for at least 15 minutes so the flaxseeds make the mixture gelatinous.

Stir dough and spread ⅛ to ¼ inches thick on parchment, plastic, or teflex dehydrator sheets.

Using a spatula, score the dough into the size crackers you want.

Dehydrate at 105° F for 8–10 hours.

Grain-free Vegan Herb Crackers

Finding a good healthy cracker can be hard. These vegan crackers are the solution! Impeccably seasoned and perfectly crunchy, they pair great with organic cheese, soup, veggies, dips, or are tasty just on their own.

2 cups almond flour

¾ teaspoon Himalayan sea salt

2 tablespoons Herbes de Provence

1 tablespoon olive oil

2 tablespoons water

MAKES 20 CRACKERS

Directions

In a large bowl, combine almond flour, salt, and Herbes de Provence. In a medium bowl, whisk together olive oil and water. Stir wet ingredients into almond flour mixture until thoroughly combined.

Roll the dough into a ball and press between 2 sheets of parchment paper to ⅛ inch thickness. Remove top piece of parchment paper.

Transfer the bottom piece with rolled out dough onto a baking sheet. Cut dough into 2-inch squares with a knife or pizza cutter.

Bake at 350° F for 9–11 minutes, until lightly golden. Let crackers cool on baking sheet for 20 minutes then serve.

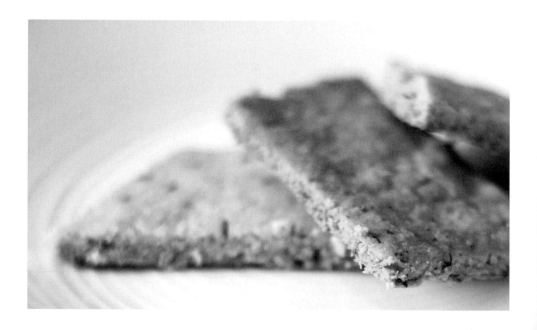

Almond Cookies

This is a quick, tasty recipe made with no flour, making it a great gluten-free dessert option.

½ teaspoon baking soda

1 teaspoon vanilla extract

⅛ – ¼ cup xylitol

1 cup almond meal

1 organic, pasture-raised egg

½ teaspoon grated lemon peel

MAKES 15 COOKIES

Directions

Preheat oven to 350° F and grease cookie sheet with grapeseed oil. Stir together almond meal, xylitol, and baking soda in a medium bowl. Add beaten egg and vanilla extract and mix well. Shape dough into balls one inch apart on cookie sheet. Bake until puffed and golden, about 10 minutes. Cool cookies on baking sheet about 2 minutes before transferring to a rack or waxed paper to cool.

> **TIP** For another variation, drizzle with melted unsweetened chocolate with stevia or xylitol added to taste.

Almond Flour Flax Meal Pizza Dough

Finally — a pizza dough that you can prepare, eat, and savor without feeling guilty or bloated, or both! This dough is also the perfect gluten-free base for paleo pizza creations, too. Top it with your favorite "maximized" pizza ingredients.

1 ¼ cups almond flour

¼ cup ground flax meal

¼ – ½ teaspoon Himalayan sea salt

¼ teaspoon aluminum free baking soda

1 organic, pasture-raised egg, beaten with a whisk

1 tablespoon extra virgin olive oil

1 teaspoon seasoning of choice – Italian seasoning or roasted garlic powder (optional)

Directions

Mix all ingredients together until they form a ball.

Roll the dough into a ¼ inch pizza crust on a sheet pan with a silpat liner or piece of parchment paper.

To make this easier, top the dough with another piece of parchment paper when you roll it out; then peel off the parchment paper when you have it the way you want it.

Bake at 350° F for 10–15 minutes.

MAKES 1 CRUST

Garlic Parmesan Flaxseed Crackers

These crackers smell great, taste good, and provide that crunch we all crave. These giant crackers can be broken down into smaller pieces and served with hummus or other dips.

1 cup flaxseed meal

⅓ cup organic Italian organic parmesan cheese, grated

1 teaspoon garlic powder

½ teaspoon Himalayan sea salt

½ cup water

SERVES 4

Directions

Preheat oven to 400° F.

Mix all the dry ingredients together, add the water, and mix. This forms a ball of dough which you can form into a rectangular disc and place on a silicone baking pad or greased parchment paper* in the middle of a cookie sheet.

Spoon onto sheet pan which is covered with a silicone mat or greased parchment paper.

Cover the mixture with a piece of parchment or waxed paper. Even out the mixture to about ⅛ inch. Use a rolling pin to level out the dough. Ensure it isn't too thin around the edges. After the mixture is spread out, push the thin edges inwards with your fingers to even it out.

Bake until the center is no longer soft, about 15–18 minutes. If it starts to get more than a little brown around the edges, remove from oven. Let cool completely – it will continue to crisp up.

Break into pieces.

*** If you don't have a silicone pad,** place the dough on a sheet of parchment paper big enough to cover the cookie sheet. Cover the dough with another sheet of parchment big enough to cover the cookie sheet. Roll out the dough between the two sheets with the rolling pin until it is approximately ⅛ of an inch thick. The rolled product should fill nearly all of the cookie sheet. Remove the top sheet of parchment and bake at 400° F for 15 to 17 minutes.

TIP Sometimes, when the outer edges are beginning to brown, the middle is not quite done. Once the giant cracker has cooled, take the softer middle of the cracker and put it back in the turned-off oven. This helps to dry the middle so it will be nice and crunchy.

Blueberry Muffins

These blueberry muffins will curb your carb craving and fill you up with real nutrients at the same time! These delicious muffins are perfect for a snack or an on-the-go breakfast that won't disappoint.

½ cup coconut flour, sifted

½ teaspoon Himalayan sea salt

½ teaspoon baking soda

6 organic, pasture-raised eggs

Stevia to taste

⅓ cup grapeseed oil

1 tablespoon vanilla extract

1 cup blueberries, fresh or frozen

MAKES 12 MUFFINS

Directions

In a small bowl, combine coconut flour, salt, and baking soda.

In a large bowl, combine eggs, grapeseed oil, and vanilla and blend well with a hand mixer.

Mix dry ingredients into wet, blending with a hand mixer.

Gently fold in blueberries.

Place batter in paper lined muffin tins.

Bake at 350° F for 20–25 minutes.

Cool and serve.

Maximized Grainless Rolls

These grainless rolls are a healthy replacement for hamburger buns or dinner rolls. They are 100% grain-free and sugar-free, so they're ideal anytime someone is looking for a bread or carb fix! You can also freeze these buns for later.

1 ½ cups almond flour

5 tablespoons psyllium husk powder

2 teaspoons aluminum-free baking powder

1 teaspoon Himalayan sea salt

2 tablespoons apple cider vinegar

2 organic, pasture-raised eggs or 3 egg whites

1 cup boiling water

Directions

Mix all of the dry ingredients together.

Add the eggs and apple cider vinegar and mix well.

Add the boiling water and continue to mix until well combined. It will turn into a very sticky dough.

Split the mixture into 5 rolls. Form into nicely shaped rolls and place them on a parchment lined baking sheet.

Bake for 50 minutes at 350° F.

MAKES 4 BURGER-SIZED BUNS

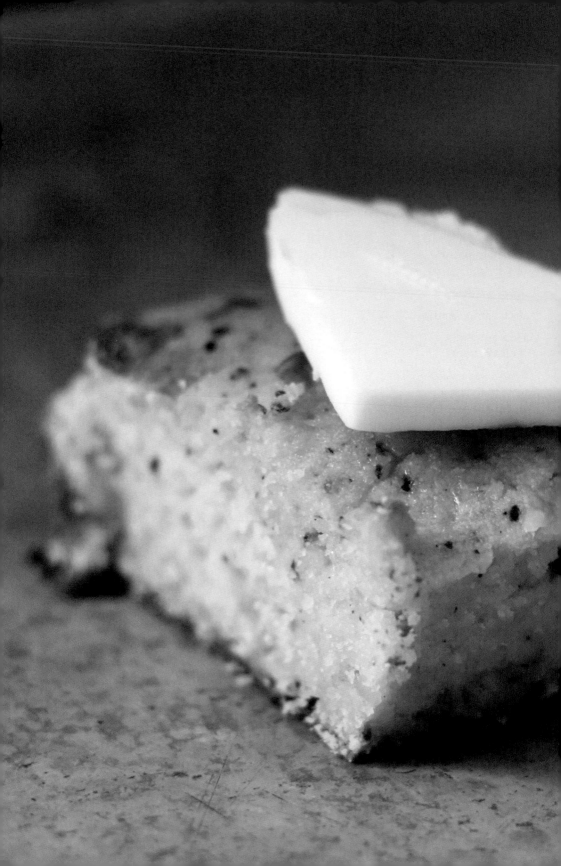

Cheesy Garlic Coconut Flour Bread

This cheesy garlic bread makes the perfect side for so many weekday meals, especially roasted vegetable lasagna or basic chili. Coconut flour works as a great substitute for traditional flour, and has more health benefits without sacrificing taste. This side dish is perfect for your next dinner party or get-together.

6 organic, pasture-raised eggs

½ cup organic butter, melted

½ teaspoon Himalayan sea salt

¾ cup coconut flour

Ground black pepper, to taste

Flaxseeds (optional), to taste

½ – 1 teaspoon garlic powder (adjust to taste)

½ – 1 cup shredded raw organic cheese

Directions

Preheat the oven to 350° F.

Blend all ingredients except cheese in a food processor until there are no lumps. If the batter is a little dry, just add a tablespoon of water as needed. It should be a moist, almost pourable batter. Stir in cheese. Pour into greased bread pan.

Bake in preheated oven for 40 minutes or until done (toothpick inserted in center comes out clean).

MAKES 1 LOAF

Carrot Cake Muffins

Many classic carrot cake muffin recipes are loaded with grains and sugars.
This healthier version tastes great, and can be quickly prepared in a food processor.

2 cups almond flour

½ teaspoon Himalayan sea salt

2 teaspoons aluminum-
free baking powder

1 tablespoon cinnamon

½ – ¾ teaspoon powdered
concentrate stevia

¼ – ½ teaspoon freshly grated nutmeg

1 scant pinch of cloves

½ cup melted organic butter

1 tablespoon vanilla (sugar-
free — check the label)

½ cup unsweetened vanilla almond
milk (or water or organic whole milk)

4 extra large or 5 large organic,
pasture-raised eggs

1 ½ cups grated organic carrots

½ cup chopped raw pecans or walnuts

Directions

Put flour, salt, baking powder, cinnamon, stevia, nutmeg, and cloves into a food processor to combine.

Add butter, vanilla, almond milk, and eggs.

Process all ingredients to combine into a slightly wet batter.

Pour the batter into a bowl over the carrots and walnuts. Stir to mix.

Divide into 12 muffin cups lined with paper or silicone liners.

Bake at 350° F for 25–30 minutes.

MAKES 12 MUFFINS

Cranberry Nut Bread

This sweet bread will add flavor and crunch to your breakfast routine or is great to use in a more savory setting. Either way, you'll have a hard time stopping at one slice.

½ cup coconut flour

1 teaspoon Himalayan sea salt

1 teaspoon baking soda

6 organic, pasture-raised eggs

½ cup grapeseed oil

Stevia, to taste

1 tablespoon vanilla extract

1 cup frozen cranberries

½ cup walnuts, chopped

Directions

In a medium bowl, combine coconut flour, salt, and baking soda.

In a large bowl, blend eggs, grapeseed oil, stevia, and vanilla.

Blend dry ingredients into wet, then fold in cranberries and walnuts.

Pour batter into two greased 6.5 × 4 inch loaf pans.

Bake at 350° F for 35 minutes.

Cool and serve.

MAKES 1 LOAF

Dark Rye Bread

Use this rye bread for anything you'd use traditional bread for, including sandwiches and croutons. This bread will pair well with your favorite soup recipes.

2 cups blanched almond flour

1 ½ cups ground flax meal

1 teaspoon Himalayan sea salt

1 teaspoon baking soda

1 ½ teaspoons cream of tartar

6 organic, pasture-raised eggs

¼ cup olive oil

½ cup water

4 tablespoons caraway seeds

Directions

Preheat oven to 350° F.

Grease a loaf pan with olive oil or coconut oil. You can add a piece of parchment for easy removal after baking.

Mix dry ingredients in one bowl except for caraway seeds.

Mix wet ingredients in another bowl.

Stir wet ingredients into the dry ones, then mix in caraway seeds.

Allow batter to sit for 1 or 2 minutes to thicken.

Pour the batter into the loaf pan, and bake for 50–60 minutes. Cool and serve.

MAKES 1 LOAF

Chocolate Zucchini Bread

The ultimate way to disguise zucchini with chocolate and bread! The zucchini makes this bread moist and guests will love it. Back off the cacao powder to create more of an everyday bread and less of a diner-like baked good.

2 ½ cups blanched almond flour (not almond meal)

½ cup cacao powder

½ teaspoon Himalayan sea salt

1 teaspoon baking soda

4 large organic, pasture-raised eggs

4 tablespoons coconut oil, room temperature

½ teaspoon vanilla stevia

1 ½ cups zucchini, grated and drained/squeezed to dry out

½ cup chopped walnuts (optional)

MAKES 1 LOAF

Directions

In a food processor combine almond flour and cacao powder.

Pulse in salt and baking soda. Pulse in eggs, coconut oil, and stevia.

Briefly pulse in zucchini. (Add 1/2 cup walnuts now if you prefer.)

Transfer batter to a greased 6.5 x 4 inch medium loaf pan, dusted with almond flour.

Bake at 350° for 35-40 minutes.

Cool for 2 hours and then serve.

Flax Meal Bread

Staying away from refined carbohydrates like bread is often difficult because they are a common staple in most people's diet. This is a healthy, crunchy alternative.

1 cup flaxseed meal

1 tablespoon aluminum-free baking powder

1 teaspoon Himalayan sea salt

1 tablespoon spoonable stevia (optional to taste)

5 organic, pasture-raised eggs, beaten

½ cup water

⅓ cup grapeseed oil or coconut oil

Directions

Preheat oven to 350° F. Prepare pan or a half-sheet pan with parchment paper or a silicone mat. Mix dry ingredients with a whisk. Mix wet ingredients; add to dry, combining well. Let batter set for 2–3 minutes to thicken up. Pour batter onto pan. Bake for about 20 minutes until it springs back when you touch the top and/or is visibly browning. Cool and cut into whatever size slices you desire.

MAKES 1 LOAF

Entrées

Roasted Vegetable Lasagna

Grass-fed Beef Squash Casserole

Asian Turkey Lettuce Wraps

Maximized Shepherd's Pie

Fish Fry Dinner

Chickpea Sweet Potato Burgers

Grilled Chicken with Chili Pepper, Bok Choy, & Ginger

Black Bean Burgers

Basil Chicken in Coconut-Curry Sauce

Lentil Walnut Balls

Herb Butter Salmon and Asparagus

Advanced Plan "Mac" & Cheese

 Core Plan   Advanced Plan   Raw   V Vegan   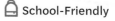 School-Friendly

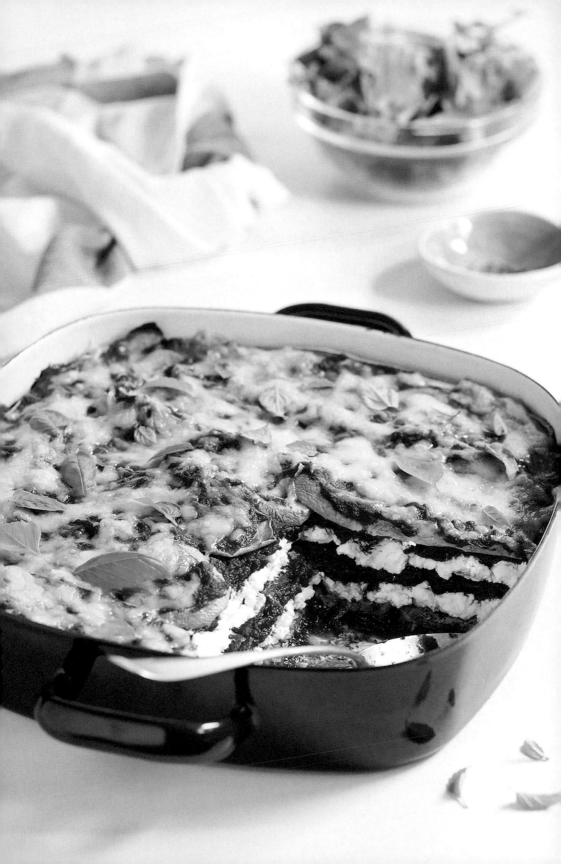

Roasted Vegetable Lasagna

This lasagna recipe takes a bit of preparation, but it is well worth the results and makes great leftovers for lunches! With no noodles, it's also gluten-free and grain-free. Serve it with a side of your favorite bread.

1 large eggplant, sliced into ¼ inch rounds

½ pound medium mushrooms, cut into ¼ inch slices

3 small zucchini, sliced lengthwise into ¼ inch slices

2 sweet red peppers, cut into 6 pieces each

3 tablespoons olive oil

1 clove garlic, minced

1 container (2 cups) organic ricotta cheese, drained

½ teaspoon ground black pepper

¼ cup organic parmesan cheese, grated

1 organic, pasture-raised egg

1 teaspoon Himalayan sea salt

3 ¼ cup pasta sauce (check ingredients for no added sugar) or homemade sauce

2 cups organic mozzarella cheese, grated

3 tablespoons basil, minced

Directions

Spread eggplant and mushrooms onto a baking pan. Place zucchini, red peppers, and onion on a second pan.

Combine oil and garlic; brush over both sides of eggplant and mushrooms.

Sprinkle with salt and pepper.

Bake uncovered at 400° F for 15 minutes.

Turn vegetables over and cook 15 minutes more. Remove eggplant and mushrooms.

Bake zucchini and red peppers for 5–10 minutes until edges are browned.

In a bowl, combine ricotta cheese, parmesan cheese, and egg.

Spread ½ cup pasta sauce in a 9 × 13 × 2 inch glass baking dish. Layer with half the ricotta cheese mixture, half of the vegetables, a third of the pasta sauce, and ⅔ cup mozzarella cheese. Sprinkle with basil. Repeat layers. Top with remaining pasta sauce.

Cover and bake at 350° F for 40 minutes.

Uncover, sprinkle with remaining cheese. Bake 5–10 minutes longer or until edges are bubbly and cheese is melted.

Let stand 10 minutes before cutting.

SERVES 4–6

Grass-fed Beef Squash Casserole

With its combination of nutrient filled grass-fed beef, squash, vegetables, and tex-mex spices, you'll be coming back to this zesty dish time and again. For a mild version, use diced green chiles instead of jalapenos. You can also use shredded cooked chicken instead of beef. Serve with your favorite side.

1 pound organic grass-fed ground beef

¼ cup coconut oil

3 organic medium zucchini, cut into ½ inch cubes

2 organic medium yellow squash, cut into ½ inch cubes

1 organic red bell pepper, chopped

1 organic jalapeño pepper, seeded and chopped

4 cloves garlic, minced

4 organic green onions, chopped — white and green ends separated

Himalayan sea salt and pepper to taste

3 tablespoons organic tomato paste

1 tablespoon chili powder (no sugar or preservatives added)

2 teaspoons ground cumin

4 cups black beans, rinsed and drained

½ cup raw organic parmesan cheese, grated and divided

¼ cup chopped fresh organic cilantro

Directions

Cook the ground beef in a stainless steel or cast iron skillet over medium heat until brown, about 10 minutes. Drain off excess grease. Set aside.

Preheat oven to 350° F.

Spread the bottom of a 9 × 13 inch baking dish with about 2 teaspoons of coconut oil.

Pour the remaining coconut oil into a large stainless steel or cast iron skillet over medium-high heat.

Cook and stir the zucchini, yellow squash, bell pepper, jalapeño pepper, garlic, and the white parts of the green onions until the vegetables begin to soften, 5–8 minutes.

Sprinkle with sea salt and black pepper. Stir in the tomato paste, chili powder, and cumin. Allow the mixture to simmer until the spices are fragrant, about 1 minute. Remove from heat.

Stir in the browned ground beef, black beans and ¼ cup of parmesan cheese until well combined. Adjust salt and pepper if necessary, and spread the mixture into the prepared baking dish. Sprinkle the top with remaining ¼ cup of parmesan cheese.

Bake in the preheated oven until bubbling in the center and cheese is browned, 20–25 minutes. Sprinkle the remaining green onions (green tops) and cilantro over the top and serve.

SERVES 8

Asian Turkey Lettuce Wraps

*This is a very tasty dish that will rival any Asian takeout or elegant restaurant.
It makes a nice presentation for an appetizer as well.*

½ cup water

3 tablespoons organic almond or cashew butter

1 pound organic ground turkey

1 tablespoon sesame oil

1 cup shiitake mushroom caps, chopped

1 tablespoon rice vinegar

1 can (1 cup) water chestnuts, drained and chopped

3 cloves garlic

2 tablespoons fresh ginger, minced

⅓ cup tamari

½ cup green onions (optional)

1 head lettuce, separated into leaves

Directions

Cook turkey in skillet about 5 minutes, stirring until turkey crumbles and is no longer pink.

Add mushrooms, rice vinegar, water chestnuts, garlic, ginger, and tamari.

Increase heat to medium-high and cook, stirring constantly, for 4 minutes.

Add green onions if desired and cook, stirring constantly, for 1 minute.

Spoon mixture evenly onto lettuce leaves; roll up. Serve with extra tamari sauce if desired.

SERVES 4–5

> **TIP** For the Core Plan, you can replace the lettuce with all natural whole wheat tortillas and also add 1/4 cup chopped carrots that have been lightly steamed.

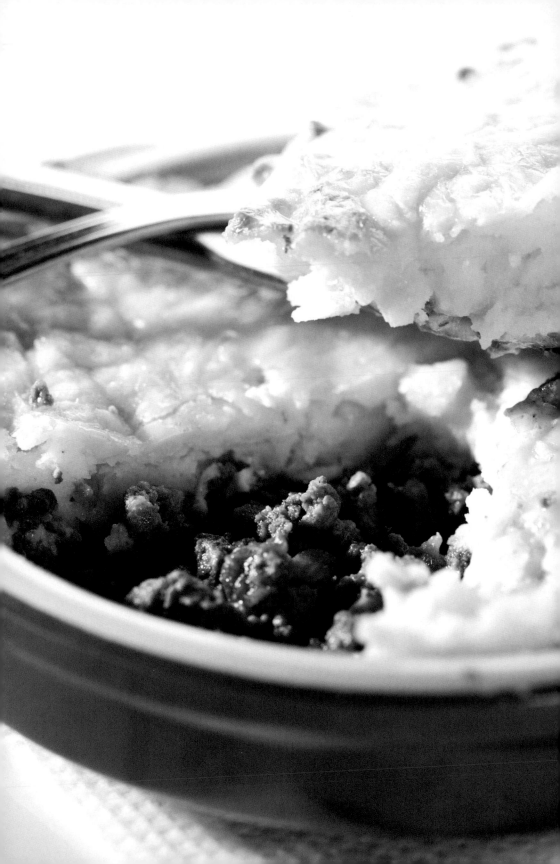

Maximized Shepherd's Pie

Shepherd's pie is a hearty favorite that can easily be transformed to fit a healthy lifestyle with this Maximized Shepherd's Pie recipe. Using Mashed NO-tatoes and your choice of ground meat, this classic comfort meal is sure to become a staple in your household.

Mashed NO-tatoes
(see page 269)

1 tablespoon coconut oil

1 large onion,
finely chopped

1 pound organic grass-
fed ground beef,
turkey, or lamb

1 stalk organic celery,
finely chopped

1 cup frozen organic peas

1 organic bell pepper,
finely chopped

1 tablespoon
arrowroot powder

2 tablespoons iced
cold water

1 cup organic
vegetable stock

2 teaspoons dried thyme

1 teaspoon dried oregano

1 pinch ground cloves

Himalayan sea salt
and pepper to taste

Directions

Prepare the *Mashed NO-tatoes* recipe and set aside.

Preheat oven to 375°F.

In a large skillet, heat the coconut oil over medium heat and add the onion and celery. Cook, stirring occasionally, until soft.

Add the ground meat, increase the heat to medium-high, and cook until browned, breaking up chunks with a wooden spoon.

Add remaining vegetables (you can add any veggies you'd like!) and sauté for 4 minutes. Add the stock, stirring to combine. Add the thyme, oregano, cloves, and sea salt and pepper.

In a small bowl, combine the arrowroot powder with the iced cold water, stirring with a fork until smooth. Add arrowroot mixture to the veggies, stirring well to combine. Bring to a boil and cook for 2–3 minutes, or until the gravy thickens. Transfer the mixture to a 9-inch round or 3-quart rectangular casserole dish.

Spread the *Mashed NO-tatoes* onto the meat mixture and spread evenly. Bake for 30–40 minutes, or until the *Mashed NO-tatoes* are golden.

SERVES 6

Fish Fry Dinner

Fried fish doesn't have to be unhealthy and with very minor changes, your children will enjoy it too! Crusting the fish in coconut flour and pan-frying it in coconut oil will give you a similar finish to your typical fish fry.

1–2 pounds of organic wild-caught fresh or frozen fish of your choice, such as flounder, grouper, red snapper, amberjack, or white fish of all varieties. You can also use thawed organic wild-caught frozen fish.

3–4 tablespoons of coconut flour

Himalayan sea salt, pepper, cayenne, lemon pepper – choose your favorite seasonings

2–3 tablespoons coconut oil

Lemon wedges (optional)

SERVES 2–4

Directions

When the rest of your dinner is prepared and your table is set, heat the coconut oil in a large skillet.

Lightly season your fish and then dust or dredge in the coconut flour.

Sauté the fish in coconut oil over medium-high heat for approximately 3–4 minutes per side, depending on the thickness of your fish, until the coating is golden brown and the fish is cooked and flakes to the touch.

Serve immediately garnished with lemon wedges (optional).

Chickpea Sweet Potato Burgers

Get creative with burger options for vegetarian and vegan guests at your summer BBQ or meatless monday dinner with these Chickpea Sweet Potato Burgers. Eat the patties alone or top them with BBQ sauce and grainless rolls. Meat lovers alike will also love this recipe!
Inspired by Paige DePaolis on Self

1 ¼ cups dried chickpeas

4 cups of water

Olive oil cooking spray

3 tablespoons tahini

¼ teaspoon freshly ground black pepper

¼ teaspoon baking powder

1 teaspoon Himalayan sea salt, divided

1 small organic sweet potato, peeled and grated

1 medium organic cucumber, peeled and thinly sliced

½ small organic red onion, thinly sliced

¼ cup chopped fresh dill

2 tablespoons rice vinegar

MAKES 4 BURGERS

Directions

In a bowl, soak chickpeas in water for at least 12 hours and up to 24 hours. Drain well.

Heat oven to 375° F. Coat a baking sheet with cooking spray.

In a food processor, process chickpeas, tahini, black pepper, baking powder, and ¾ teaspoon salt. Scrape down sides as necessary, until mixture holds together when pinched, about 2 minutes. Transfer to a bowl and stir in sweet potato.

In a second bowl, combine cucumber, onion, dill, vinegar and remaining ¼ teaspoon salt and set aside.

Form chickpea-sweet potato mixture into 4 burgers. Place on baking sheet then cover tightly with foil and bake for 20 minutes.

Remove foil. Coat burgers with spray then bake until crisp and golden underneath, about 20–25 minutes.

Flip burgers. Coat with cooking spray then bake until crisp on other side, about 10–15 minutes.

Serve with cucumber, onion, or dill mix for added flavor.

TIP If you don't have olive oil cooking spray, just pour some olive oil in a cup and spread it lightly on the burger with a pastry brush.

Grilled Chicken with Chili Pepper, Bok Choy, & Ginger

Bok Choy is a type of cabbage that offers tremendous health benefits. As the main ingredient in this healthy and tasty dish, you're receiving maximum nutrition.

1 cup organic, pasture-raised chicken breast

2 cloves fresh garlic, crushed

1 tablespoon fresh ginger, grated

1–2 tablespoons soy sauce or tamari (plus extra for serving)

1 tablespoon mirin

2 cups bok choy, sliced

2 tablespoons coconut oil

2 cups fresh shiitake or portobello mushrooms, washed and sliced

½ mild chili pepper, seeded and chopped

2 small green onions, sliced

1–2 teaspoons dark sesame oil (optional)

½ – 1 teaspoon toasted sesame seeds

Directions

Mix chicken together with half the garlic, half the ginger, soy sauce, and mirin and set aside.

Heat 1 tablespoon oil in a wok or large pot and add mushrooms, bok choy, chili pepper, green onions, and remaining garlic and ginger. Stir fry for about 6 minutes or until bok choy is tender but still crisp.

Meanwhile, brush chicken with marinade. Pick up a piece of chicken and let excess juices run off. Place the chicken on the hot grill pan and repeat with remaining chicken.

Cook for 2–3 minutes until it is seared and has brown stripes then flip pieces over to cook the other side.

Add any remaining marinade to the bok choy mixture, stir, and season with sea salt and pepper, sesame oil, and a dash of soy sauce or tamari. To serve, sprinkle with sesame seeds.

SERVES 2–4

Black Bean Burgers

Looking for the perfect meatless monday meal? These spicy sliders are tough to resist, even for your meat-loving friends. Brown these flavorful moist burger patties either on the backyard grill at a summer barbecue, indoors in a skillet for a weeknight dinner, or as an appetizer.

1 can (2 cups) organic, low-sodium black beans, drained well

1 teaspoon cumin

2 cloves garlic, minced

¼ cup green onion, sliced — reserve a few for garnish

Jalapeños, diced (optional)

1–2 tablespoons extra virgin olive oil

Lime wedges for garnish

6 *Maximized Grainless Rolls* (see page 245)

MAKES 6 PATTIES

Directions

In a medium sized mixing bowl, add black beans. With the back of a fork, smash about ¾ of the beans into a paste.

Add to the bowl cumin, garlic, green onion, and jalapenos. Form beans into 6 patties, the same diameter of your biscuits. Set aside.

Pop rolls in the oven now. Grill the grainless rolls.

In a medium sized skillet, heat olive oil over medium heat. Once hot, add bean patties and cook until browned about 5 minutes. Flip and brown the other side.

Serve immediately on grainless rolls or your bread of choice. Garnish with green onion, a lime wedge, and your choice of yogurt sauce or mayonnaise.

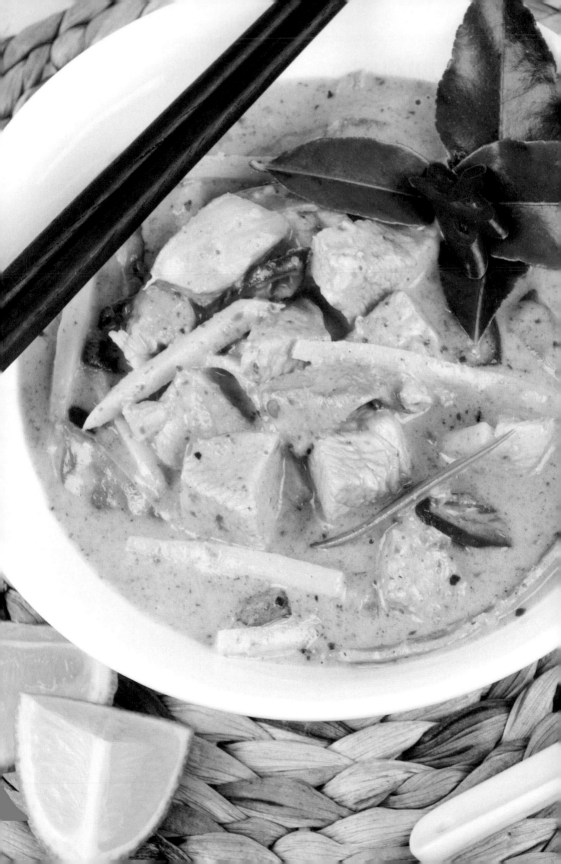

Basil Chicken in Coconut-Curry Sauce

Curry is a great way to shake up your traditional chicken dinners with spice, flavor, protein, and healthy fats. Serve it alone or with coconut lime rice, cucumber salad, or grainless rolls.

4 organic, pasture-raised, skinless, boneless chicken breasts

½ teaspoon Himalayan sea salt

½ teaspoon ground cumin

½ teaspoon ground coriander

½ teaspoon ground cloves

½ teaspoon ground cinnamon

½ teaspoon cardamom

½ teaspoon fresh black pepper

¼ teaspoon chili powder

¼ teaspoon ground turmeric

1 large red onion, diced

6 cloves garlic, minced

2 jalapeño peppers, seeded and minced

1 tablespoon coconut oil

2 cups organic, full fat coconut milk

2 teaspoons arrowroot

3 tablespoons fresh basil

1 tablespoon chopped ginger root

Directions

Rinse chicken and pat dry. Cut into 1-inch pieces and place in medium bowl.

In a small bowl, stir together all spices. Sprinkle over chicken pieces, toss to coat well. Cover and let stand at room temperature for 30 minutes or in fridge up to 2 hours.

In stainless steel skillet, heat coconut oil over medium-high heat. Add onion, garlic, and jalapeño and cook for about 2–3 minutes. Remove, reserving drippings in the skillet.

Add half of the chicken to skillet. Cook and stir for 3 minutes or until cooked through. Remove chicken and add remaining half; cook through. Remove from skillet.

Combine coconut milk with arrowroot and carefully add to skillet. Cook and stir over medium-high heat until thick and bubbly. Add chicken mixture, whole basil leaves, and ginger root. Cook 2 minutes more to heat through.

Serve over wild rice (core plan only) and garnish with red onion wedges and basil.

SERVES 4

Lentil Walnut Balls

Looking for the perfect protein-filled, tasty snack? Eat these vegan bites plain or as a side dish to any meal. They're even a great addition to your favorite salad for a plant-based main course option.

½ cup uncooked lentils

1 cup walnuts halves, finely chopped

2 teaspoons coconut oil

2 heaping cups of finely chopped cremini mushrooms

3 large cloves of garlic, minced

1 cup of kale, finely chopped, stems removed

½ teaspoon dried oregano

1 tablespoon lemon juice

2 tablespoons ground flax

3 tablespoons water

⅓ cup ground almonds

½ teaspoon Himalayan sea salt, to taste

Freshly ground black pepper, to taste

SERVES 2

Directions

Add lentils into a medium pot along with 2¼ cups water. Bring to a boil and then reduce heat to medium. Simmer for about 20 minutes, uncovered, adding more water if the lentils dry out.

Once the lentils are tender to the fork, remove from heat and mash with a potato masher into acoarse paste with some lentil pieces still intact. Set aside.

Heat oven to 350°F.

In a very large skillet, add the oil along with the finely chopped mushrooms and garlic. Season with salt. Sauté over medium-high heat for about 7–9 minutes, until most of the water cooks off.

Add kale, walnuts, herbs, and lemon juice. Stir until combined and continue cooking for another few minutes until the kale is wilted. Remove from heat and stir in the mashed lentils when ready.

In a small bowl, whisk together the ground flax and 3 tablespoons water. Stir for 10 seconds and then immediately pour into the skillet mixture. Stir to combine.

Stir in the ⅓ cup ground almond flour until combined. Season with salt and pepper to taste. The mixture should be fairly moist and sticky. If it's too sticky, add more ground almonds. If it's dry, add another tablespoon of water.

Line a baking sheet with parchment paper. Shape lentil mixture into balls and pack tightly with your hands so they hold together.

Place on baking sheet an inch or so apart. Repeat for the rest. If the mixture is too hot to handle, let it cool for a bit first and then proceed. Bake the lentil balls at 350°F for 15 minutes. Remove from oven, gently flip over, and bake for another 11–13 minutes, until golden and firm on the exterior.

Herb Butter Salmon and Asparagus

Baking asparagus and salmon together in parchment paper inside a foil pack deliciously melds together their flavors and makes for a juicy entrée.

4 organic boneless, skinless wild-caught salmon fillets

Himalayan sea salt and pepper to taste

1 pound organic asparagus, ends trimmed

1 lemon, thinly sliced (plus additional wedges for garnish)

½ cup organic butter, at room temperature

3 teaspoons Italian seasoning

3 teaspoons minced garlic

fresh thyme or parsley, for garnish (optional)

SERVES 4

Directions

Season salmon generously with salt and pepper on both sides. Arrange one salmon fillet and ¼ of the asparagus in the center of one 12 x 12 inch piece of foil. Repeat with remaining salmon and asparagus on 3 other pieces of foil. Slide lemon slices under the salmon and asparagus.

In a small bowl mix butter, Italian seasoning, and garlic. Drop large dollops of the herb butter on top of the salmon and asparagus.

Fold the parchment paper and foil tightly around the salmon and asparagus, being sure to seal the ends together tightly so the juices and butter doesn't run out while cooking.

Bake at 425°F for 30 minutes, until asparagus is tender and salmon is flaky.

Drizzle fresh lemon juice over the top and serve immediately.

Advanced Plan "Mac" & Cheese

One of your favorite comfort foods has a healthier alternative! Using the very versatile hearts of palm, this decadent recipe is quick and easy to make. This dish is sure to become a weeknight dinner staple in your household alone or with Southern-style biscuits or grainless rolls.

¼ cup organic butter

3 tablespoons organic cream cheese

¼ cup organic chicken broth

1 cup organic cheddar cheese, shredded

Himalayan sea salt and pepper, to taste

2 jars of hearts of palm

Additional organic shredded cheese (for topping)

SERVES 2–4

Directions

In a saucepan, melt butter over medium heat.

Stir in cream cheese and broth until completely combined and smooth. Reduce heat slightly and add cheddar cheese, stirring until melted.

Add salt and pepper to taste. Remove from heat.

Instead of traditional macaroni noodles, simply cut two jars of hearts of palm into discs (or moon shapes by cutting the cylinder in half lengthways then into slices) and boil in filtered water for 5–7 minutes. Drain well and add cheese sauce.

Put into a baking dish and top with cheese and bake at 350° F until bubbly.

Sides

Green Bean Amandine

Mashed NO-tatoes

Roasted Veggies

Grain-free Vegetable Nut Stuffing

 Core Plan   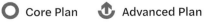 Advanced Plan   Raw   Vegan   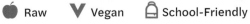 School-Friendly

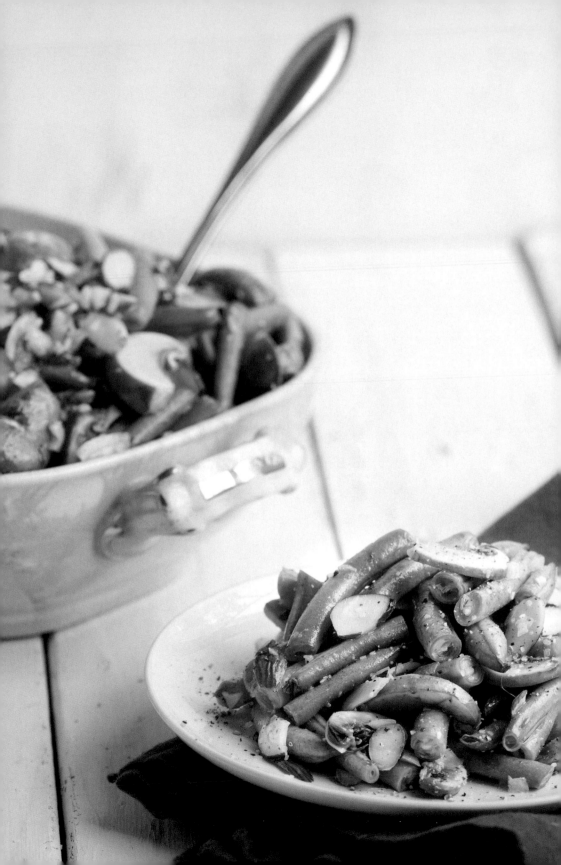

◀ Green Bean Amandine

Nutrient-rich and full of flavor, this lemony recipe will become one of your new favorite side dishes. It is simple to make, but needs to be dehydrated and chilled overnight. In this recipe, the green beans remain completely intact.

3 tablespoons lemon juice

8 tablespoons olive oil

1 clove of garlic, minced

1 tablespoon onion, minced

1/2 teaspoon dry mustard

1/2 teaspoon Himalayan sea salt

1/4 teaspoon fresh ground pepper

4 cups green beans, fresh cut

2 cups mushrooms, wiped and sliced

1 cup almonds, sliced

Directions

Combine ingredients for marinade and pour over beans, mushrooms and almonds. Toss well.

Allow to marinate for 2 hours in a dehydrator or overnight in the refrigerator.

Serve chilled or just slightly warmed.

SERVES 4

Mashed NO-tatoes

Cauliflower is a very versatile vegetable; it can do wonderful things. This Mashed No-tatoes recipe is a low-carb, nutritious, and delicious alternative to high carbohydrate mashed potatoes or a rice dish. Use this recipe for the top of your Maximized Shepherd's Pie, or serve as a side to your holiday feast or favorite casserole meal.

1 head cauliflower

2 tablespoons organic butter

1–2 cloves of garlic (optional)

Himalayan sea salt and black pepper, to taste

SERVES 4–6

Directions

Steam cauliflower until very soft.

Chop up cauliflower and put in a food processor or blender with butter, salt, pepper, and garlic if desired. Blend to desired consistency.

Serve immediately or store for later. If reheating, bake at 350°F for 25-35 minutes until these are beautifully browned.

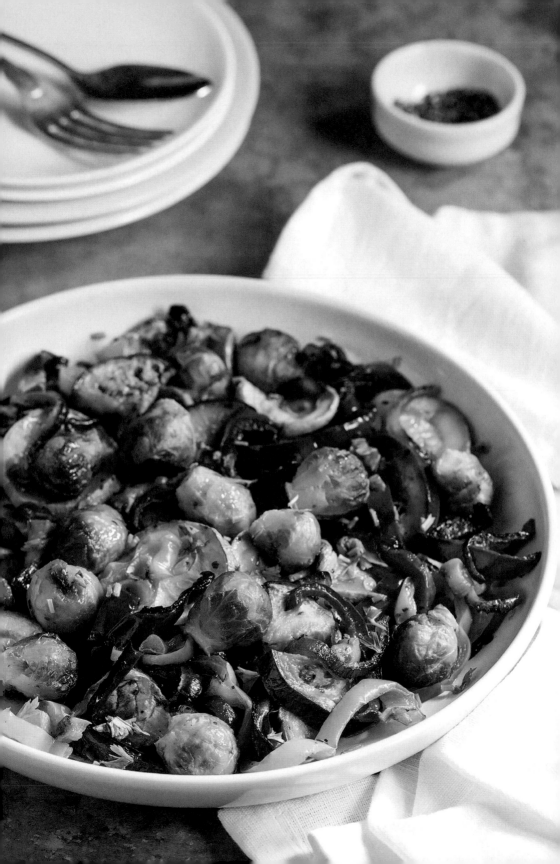

Roasted Veggies

Double up your veggie intake with this Roasted Veggies recipe. It's a healthy side dish for any dinner, holiday meal, or potluck, and can be tailored to fit whatever vegetables are in season, and also can be seasoned many different ways. If following the core plan, try mixing in carrots or sweet potatoes for extra flavor and breadth.

2 tablespoons balsamic vinegar

1 teaspoon Dijon mustard

½ cup extra-virgin olive oil

3 garlic cloves, pressed

2 teaspoons finely chopped fresh thyme (or ½ tsp dried thyme)

1 teaspoon finely chopped fresh basil (or ¼ tsp dried basil)

2 large red onions, thinly sliced

3 bell peppers (any color), sliced

1 1-pound eggplant, quartered lengthwise, cut into slices

2 organic yellow squash cut into rounds

2 organic zucchini cut into rounds

15-20 brussels sprouts (cut larger ones in half)

Himalayan sea salt to taste

Directions

Whisk vinegar and mustard in medium bowl. Gradually whisk in oil.

Stir in garlic, thyme, and basil and season to taste with salt and pepper.

Preheat oven to 450°F.

Toss vegetables with the dressing; toss to coat.

Divide between 2 large rimmed baking sheets.

Roast until vegetables are tender and slightly brown around edges, about 35 minutes.

SERVES 2–4

Grain-free Vegetable Nut Stuffing ○ ⟱

Here's a great stuffing option for your feast! This recipe contains no grains, but is packed with protein and healthy fats. It can be made with or without meat as preferred. The addition of nuts and seeds give the dish a nice crunchy flavor that everyone is sure to enjoy.

½ large sweet (vidalia) onion, coarsely chopped

1 large bulb fennel (white part only) cut in half, then cut lengthwise into ¼ inch-wide strips

4–5 stalks celery (including leaves), chopped

¼ cup extra virgin olive oil

1 cup organic chicken broth

½ teaspoon rubbed sage

¼ teaspoon oregano

½ –1 cup chopped walnuts (optional)

½ cup raw sunflower seeds (soaked if possible)

1 cup mushrooms, chopped

Himalayan sea salt and ground pepper, to taste

2 tablespoons chopped fresh parsley

½ –1 pound organic ground turkey, organic turkey sausage, or organic chicken sausage, crumbled and cooked on the stovetop (optional)

SERVES 2–4

Directions

Heat oil in a deep sauté pan. Add onions, fennel and celery. Heat on medium for several minutes until vegetables are lightly browned.

Add chicken stock, bring to a boil, reduce heat to low and cover pan. Simmer ingredients for 20 minutes.

Add sage, oregano and salt and pepper to taste. Add walnuts and sunflower seeds, cover and continue to cook mixture, stirring occasionally, for 5 minutes.

Add mushrooms and meat (if desired), cover and cook on medium for an additional 10–12 minutes, stirring occasionally.

If there is excess liquid, cook uncovered to reduce. If the mixture is too dry, add more chicken stock, a little bit at a time.

Check seasonings and add additional salt and pepper if needed. Sprinkle with chopped parsley.

Sauces, Dips & Dressings

All-Natural Barbecue Sauce

Nine Layer Taco Dip

Caesar Salad Dressing

Taco Seasoning Mix

Spicy Cashew Mayo

Raw Vegan Ranch Sauce

Chili Lime Salad Dressing

Garlic White Bean Dip

Classic Hummus

Zesty Walnut Hummus

Sundried Tomato Hummus

Baba Ganoush

Puttanesca Salsa

Healing Turmeric Dressing

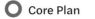 Core Plan   Advanced Plan   Raw    Vegan   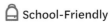 School-Friendly

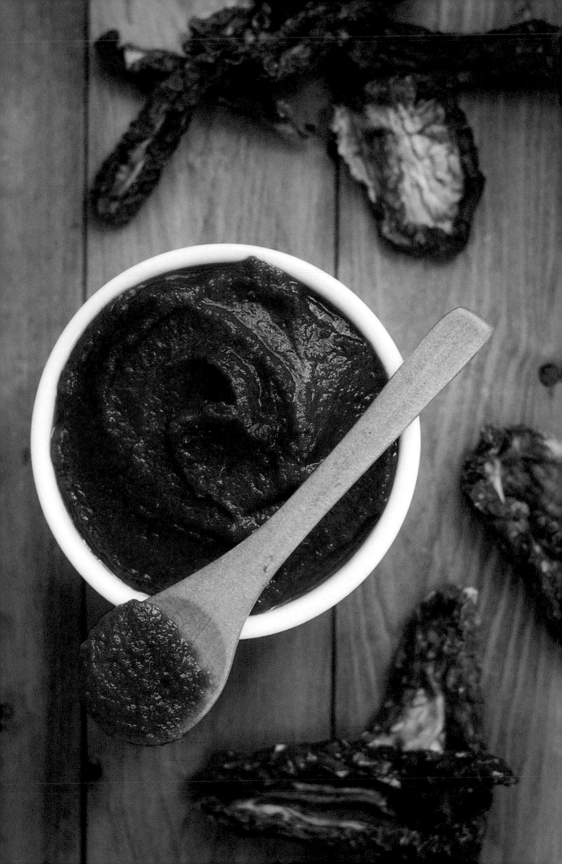

All-Natural Barbecue Sauce

This barbecue sauce has no added sugars or artificial sweeteners—just the natural sweetness of dates.

40g sun-dried tomatoes (soaked overnight)

120g dates (soaked overnight)

1 teaspoon olive oil

40g chopped onion

1 small garlic clove

2 medium roasted tomatoes

1 tablespoon tamari sauce (double-check for wheat if avoiding gluten)

1 teaspoon lime juice

2 teaspoons smoked paprika

1/4 teaspoon smoked Chipotle powder (optional for a spicy sauce)

Liquid smoke (optional for a hickory flavor — be sure to use a brand that is concentrated hickory without molasses or artificial ingredients)

Directions

Soak the sun-dried tomatoes in 1/2 cup of clean water, and dates in 1 cup of clean water overnight. Keep all of the soaking water for blending.

Wash the fresh tomatoes and put in the oven at 350°F until the skin turns dark (about 45-60 minutes). Rotate them a couple of times. Let cool, peel the skin off and remove the seeds.

Heat the olive oil in a saucepan. Add the chopped onion and garlic, and cook until they turn brown.

Combine all the ingredients in a blender. It should be fairly liquid and easy to blend. If its too thick, add a little more water until it blends easily.

Put the previous mixture in a sauce pan and cook at low heat until the water starts to evaporate and the sauce gets more dense. Put back in the blender to make it a little more homogeneous if needed.

MAKES 1 SMALL JAR

Nine Layer Taco Dip

Is it game day? Are you having a party? Either way, this nine layer taco dip will have everyone hovering around the snack table! A widespread mix of layered vegetables perfectly paired with a combination of spices, cheese, and beans takes this nine layer dip to the next level of party food. Serve it with organic flaxseed crackers and fresh organic vegetables.

Seasoning Mix

3 tablespoons chili powder

1 teaspoon garlic powder

3 teaspoons ground cumin

1 ½ teaspoon paprika

2 teaspoons oregano

1 teaspoon onion powder

½ teaspoon cayenne pepper, or to taste

½ teaspoon Himalayan sea salt

2 teaspoons black pepper

The Layers

1 can organic refried black beans

1 cup organic cream cheese, softened

2 cups organic sour cream

2 cups organic salsa

1 large organic tomato, chopped

1 organic green bell pepper, chopped

1 bunch organic green onions, chopped

1 heart organic romaine lettuce, shredded

¾ cup sliced black olives

2 avocados, diced

Squeeze of lime juice

2 cups raw cheddar cheese, shredded

Directions

In a medium bowl, blend the taco seasoning mix and refried beans together. Spread the mixture onto a large serving platter.

Mix the sour cream and cream cheese in a medium bowl. Spread over the refried beans. Top the layers with salsa.

Place a layer of tomato, green bell pepper, green onions, and lettuce over the salsa, and top with cheddar cheese.

In a small bowl, mix the diced avocado with lime juice.

Garnish the layers with black olives and avocado.

SERVES 12

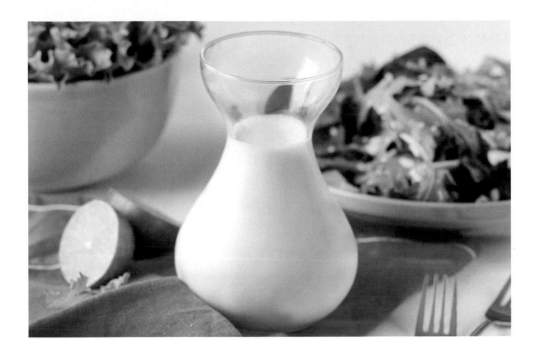

Caesar Salad Dressing

This dressing comes together quickly and is a tasty, healthy substitute for traditional store-bought dressing. Turn your salad into a meal by adding turkey bacon, old fashioned BBQ chicken, or spiced grass-fed beef roast. For best results, chill before using.

1 organic, pasture-raised egg

½ cup white wine vinegar

2 tablespoons lemon juice

2 garlic cloves

½ teaspoon Himalayan sea salt

¼ teaspoon pepper

¾ cup olive oil

⅓ cup freshly grated raw organic parmesan cheese

Directions

In a blender or food processor, add all ingredients besides olive oil. Blend well.

While the processor is running, gradually add in the olive oil – it should take you several minutes to add all the oil.

Use immediately or refrigerate for up to 1 week.

MAKES 2 CUPS

Taco Seasoning Mix

Making your own seasonings is very easy and so much healthier than the kind you buy in a package. This homemade seasoning doesn't include any artificial ingredients or additives.

2 tablespoons chili powder

½ teaspoon onion powder

2 tablespoons flour (optional)

½ teaspoon garlic powder

½ teaspoon Himalayan sea salt

2 teaspoons oregano

2 teaspoons cumin

½ teaspoon cayenne pepper

Directions

Combine all ingredients in a ziplock bag and shake until completely mixed.

Add to browned ground beef or your favorite vegetarian alternative along with 1/2–3/4 cup water and cook until reduced to desired consistency.

**MAKES ENOUGH FOR
1 POUND OF MEAT**

Spicy Cashew Mayo

This mayo is plant-based and delicious. Use this spicy topping on your favorite salad, sandwich, or black bean slider. It tastes amazing as a dip for sweet potato wedges or on a party platter!

2 cups cashews, pre-soaked for 2 hours

4 tablespoons apple cider vinegar

4 tablespoons organic red miso paste

2 tablespoons Dijon mustard

6-8 tablespoons water

Directions

Put all ingredients in a high-speed blender such as a BlendTec® or Vitamix®. Blend on high speed until smooth.

Refrigerate and serve.

MAKES 2 CUPS

Raw Vegan Ranch Sauce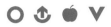

This is the simplest, tastiest, and healthiest vegan ranch sauce recipe you'll ever find. You will need a high speed blender such as a Vitamix® or Blendtec® to make it, but after that you only need 5 minutes, some cashews, and an appetite.

1 ¼ cups raw cashews

¾ cup water or coconut water

3 tablespoons lemon juice

¼ cup apple cider vinegar

⅓ cup extra virgin olive oil

2 cloves garlic

3 teaspoons onion powder

1 teaspoon dried dill

1 teaspoon Himalayan sea salt

Directions

Put everything into a high speed blender. Blend until creamy.

If needed, add more water.

SERVES 8-10

Chili Lime Salad Dressing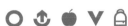

This salad dressing is an easy twist on a typical balsamic vinegar and olive oil dressing. This recipe takes about 3 minutes to prepare and lasts for a week or two.

½ cup freshly squeezed lime juice

1 cup extra virgin olive oil

½ teaspoon Himalayan sea salt

½ teaspoon Mexican chili powder

1 or 2 cloves garlic, minced
or grated into the mix

Directions

Pour all the ingredients into a resealable jar and shake vigorously.

SERVES 4-6

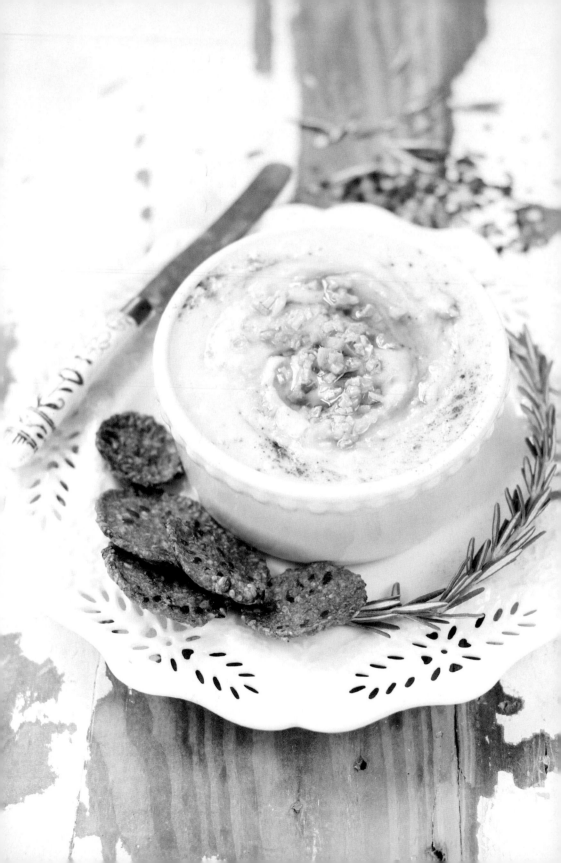

Garlic White Bean Dip

This quick and simple dip is the perfect appetizer for your next potluck or party. Just a few ingredients deliver a flavorful dip that guests will swoon for! Serve with fresh veggies or savory flax crackers for a tasty starter or serve this cold with crackers and watch as it's eaten up!

½ tablespoon oil
for cooking

4–5 cloves garlic, peeled
and finely minced

2 cups white beans
(cannellini), preferably
freshly cooked

1 tablespoon freshly
squeezed lemon juice

1 tablespoon water

1 tablespoon olive oil

½ teaspoon cumin

½ teaspoon
rosemary powder

Pinch of hot paprika
or red chili pepper

Himalayan sea salt and
black pepper, to taste

Directions

Add the cooking oil to a small skillet over medium–low heat. Sweat garlic for about 2 minutes or until light gold in color. Be careful not to brown or burn the garlic or it will turn bitter. Set aside.

Combine all remaining ingredients in a food processor and blend until smooth. Add another tablespoon of water if the dip appears to be too dry.

Add roasted garlic to your dip and pulse, or top your dip with the roasted garlic and serve with vegetable sticks or crackers.

SERVES 4–6

Classic Hummus

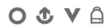

This unique dressing contains anti-inflammatory superfoods real stalks of turmeric and ginger, apple cider vinegar, garlic, and extra virgin olive oil. Feel free to play with the quantities of each ingredient, to taste. Use it on any salad or as a dip for your favorite snacks. This versatile dressing pairs well with many ingredients in salads such as fish, vegetables, and more.

1 can chickpeas

2 tablespoons reserved liquid from chickpeas

2 cloves garlic, pressed or minced

Juice of 1 lemon

3 tablespoons extra virgin olive oil

1–2 tablespoons of tahini (sesame paste)

Himalayan sea salt

Optional ingredients

Fresh parsley, paprika, cumin, cayenne pepper

Directions

Put chickpeas, reserved liquid, lemon juice, salt, tahini, and garlic in a food processor and blend until smooth.

Slowly add the olive oil. You can add more or less to reach your desired consistency.

SERVES 4–6

Zesty Walnut Hummus

Try this tasty twist on a classic snack that packs a nourishing punch of omega-3 fatty acids. Couple this easy-to-prepare, creamy dip with grain-free crackers or fresh veggies to create the perfect snack or appetizer.

½ cup walnuts, toasted

1 can (2 ⅓ cups) chickpeas, drained and rinsed

¼ cup Italian salad dressing (lemon juice, olive oil, and Italian seasoning)

½ teaspoon cayenne pepper

Directions

In a blender or food processor, purée walnuts, chickpeas, salad dressing, and cayenne pepper together until smooth.

Serve with vegetables or crackers.

SERVES 4–6

Sundried Tomato Hummus

○ ⚓ V 🔒

Sundried tomato and basil put a delicious twist on traditional hummus. Packed with flavor, fiber and nutrients, this sundried tomato hummus is sure to be a crowd-pleaser at your next party or become your new favorite go-to snack. Serve with fresh vegetables or crackers.

4 cloves of garlic

1 teaspoon Himalayan sea salt

¼ cup fresh lemon juice

2 cans (15.5 ounces) of chickpeas, drained and rinsed

½ cup olive oil

½ cup sundried tomatoes

¼ cup fresh finely chopped basil

2 teaspoons cumin

1 tablespoons sriracha hot sauce (optional)

Directions

Place garlic, salt, and lemon juice in processor. Process until smooth.

Pour in the chickpeas and ½ cup olive oil. Process until smooth again, scraping the sides of the bowl.

Once smooth, add the sundried tomatoes and pulse until they have been chopped to very small pieces and are incorporated into the hummus.

Add the basil and pulse few times until mixed in.

SERVES 6-8

Baba Ganoush

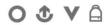

This traditional Middle Eastern eggplant dip is very impressive in taste and presentation without a lot of fuss. Pair it with raw vegetables for a tasty healthy snack.

2 globe eggplants
(about 2 pounds)

3 tablespoons extra
virgin olive oil

2 tablespoons tahini
(sesame paste)

1 clove garlic, finely
minced or pressed

½ teaspoon ground cumin

2 ½ tablespoons lemon
juice, freshly squeezed

¾ teaspoon
Himalayan sea salt

Cayenne pepper, to taste

1 tablespoon
cilantro, chopped

Directions

Preheat the oven to 375°F.

Cut the eggplant in half lengthwise and brush with olive oil. Place on a baking sheet, cut side down and roast until very tender, about 35 minutes.

Place the eggplant in a colander to drain and cool for 15 minutes, then scoop the flesh out of the skin.

Combine the eggplant, remaining olive oil, tahini, garlic, cumin, 2 tablespoons of the lemon juice, the salt, and a pinch of cayenne in the work bowl of a food processor. Pulse until the eggplant is smooth but retains some of its texture.

Allow the baba ganoush to sit for one hour at room temperature, then season it to taste with additional lemon juice, salt, and cayenne. Toss in cilantro and serve with raw vegetables.

SERVES 4–6

Puttanesca Salsa

This salsa can be used many ways — over fish, chicken, or lamb; as an ingredient in an organic sour cream dip; or tossed with zucchini noodles or cauliflower "rice." You will no doubt think of other ways to use it once you taste this highly flavorful and extremely versatile salsa. No cooking required!

1 ½ teaspoons anchovy paste

2–3 cloves garlic, grated

1 teaspoon crushed red pepper flakes

1 lemon, zested and juiced

3 tablespoons capers, chopped if necessary

½ cup pitted black olives, chopped

½ cup flat-leaf parsley, coarsely chopped

1 pint grape tomatoes, halved, or cherry tomatoes, quartered

¼ cup extra virgin olive oil

Directions

In the bottom of a medium bowl, combine anchovy paste, grated garlic, red pepper flakes, zest and lemon juice.

Whisk in ¼ cup olive oil.

Add capers, olives, parsley, and tomatoes.

Toss and season with black pepper (optional).

Serve immediately or refrigerate for up to 5 days.

SERVES 3–4

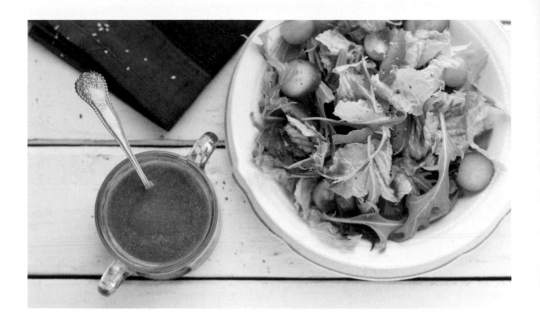

Healing Turmeric Dressing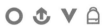

This unique dressing contains anti-inflammatory superfoods real stalks of turmeric and ginger, apple cider vinegar, garlic, and extra virgin olive oil. Feel free to play with the quantities of each ingredient, to taste. Use it on any salad or as a dip for your favorite snacks. This versatile dressing pairs well with many ingredients in salads such as fish, vegetables, and more.

1 cup extra virgin olive oil

¼ cup apple cider vinegar

3–4 cloves garlic

One inch of ginger

3 inches of turmeric

1 teaspoon balsamic vinegar

Liquid stevia, to taste

Directions

Chop an inch off the garlic and 3 inches off the turmeric, and put it in the blender.

Churn all ingredients up in the blender.

Serve cooled on your favorite salad or with your favorite snacks. If you are bringing it to work with you, make sure to keep the salad and the dressing separate until you eat!

SERVES 4–6

Desserts

Apple Berry Crisp

Strawberry Gelato

Chocolate Mousse

Sugar-free Cinnabites

Almond Flour Lemon Bars

Whole Food Date Caramels

Grain-free Chocolate Cupcakes

Primal Pots de Crème

Raw Brownie Balls

Black-Bottom Strawberry Pie

Cinnamon Spice Pecans

Vegan Vanilla Ice Cream

Almond Butter Cups

Chocolate Truffles

Chocolate Chunk Brownies

 Core Plan Advanced Plan 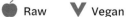 Raw V Vegan School-Friendly

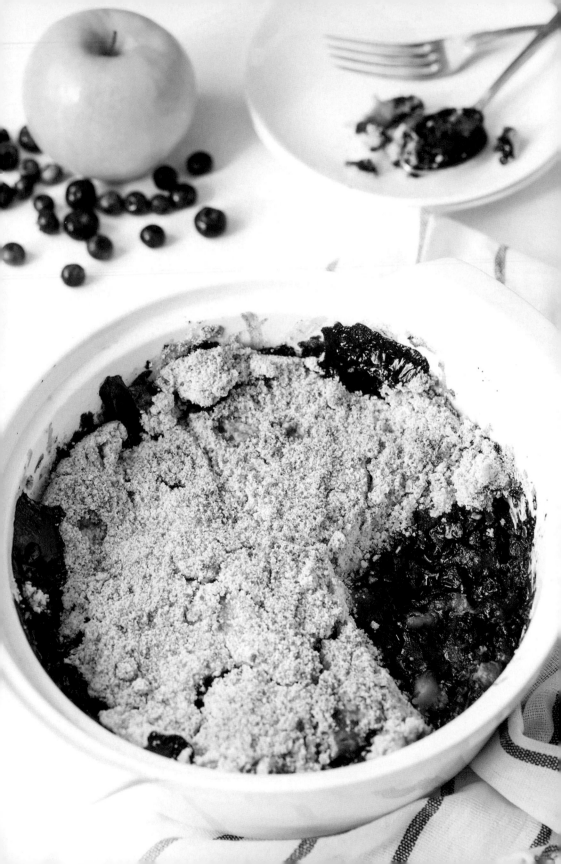

Apple Berry Crisp

This delicious recipe gives you the healthy benefits of antioxidants and dietary fiber from apples and berries. Add a side of ice cream of your choosing, or top it with whipped cream — though it tastes just as great without additions.

5 (preferably organic) granny smith apples, peeled, cored, and chopped into bite sized pieces

1 pint fresh blackberries (or your favorite berries)

1 tablespoon lemon juice

1 tablespoon pure vanilla extract (sugar-free — check the label)

2 tablespoons blanched almond flour

1 cup blanched almond flour

¼ teaspoon Himalayan sea salt

¼ teaspoon baking soda

2 ½ tablespoons olive oil

SERVES 2–4

Directions

Place apples and berries in a large bowl.

Sprinkle with lemon juice, vanilla, and 2 tablespoons blanched almond flour, tossing to incorporate all ingredients.

Place apple-berry mixture in an 8 × 8 inch baking dish and set aside.

To assemble the topping, in a medium bowl, combine almond flour, salt, baking soda, and oil.

Crumble the topping over apple-berry mixture.

Cover with tinfoil and bake at 350° F for 60–75 minutes until fruit is juicy and bubbling.

Remove from oven and uncover.

If topping is lightly browned, allow to cool for 10–15 minutes. If topping is not yet browned, place in oven uncovered for 5 minutes, or until lightly browned.

Serve warm or cold.

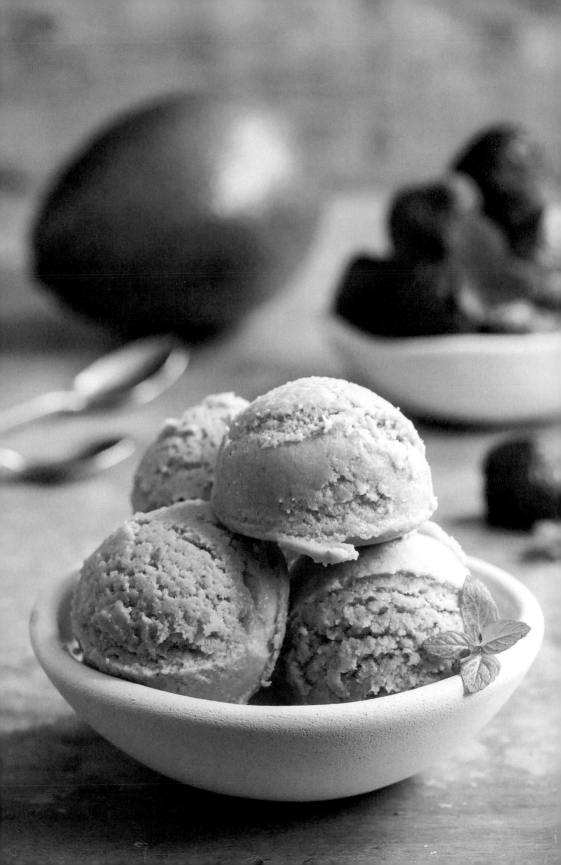

◀ Strawberry Gelato

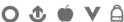

Beat the heat in the summer with this delicious and refreshing gelato recipe, or serve it as an after-school treat. Just three simple ingredients will make this dessert one of your favorite cool treats!

2 cups of frozen organic strawberries

1 ripe avocado, pit and peel removed

Stevia to taste

Directions

Put the strawberries and avocado in a heavy duty blender (preferably with a plunger).

Make sure you blend it well then add stevia to taste.

SERVES 2–4

Chocolate Mousse

You won't believe how rich, smooth, and delicious this recipe is. The surprise ingredient: avocados! This chocolate mousse is great alone or served as a fondue with fresh strawberries, bananas, or tangerines.

½ cup medjool dates, soaked

Stevia, to taste

1 teaspoon vanilla extract (optional)

3 mashed avocados

¾ cup organic cocoa

½ cup water

Directions

Place the dates, stevia, and vanilla extract in a food processor and process until smooth.

Add the mashed avocado and cocoa powder and process until creamy. You may need to stop and scrape down the sides of the bowl with a spatula a few times.

Add the water and process until smooth.

Serve at room temperature or chilled.

Store in a sealed container in the refrigerator. Chocolate mousse will keep up to 3 days in the refrigerator and 2 weeks in the freezer.

SERVES 3–4

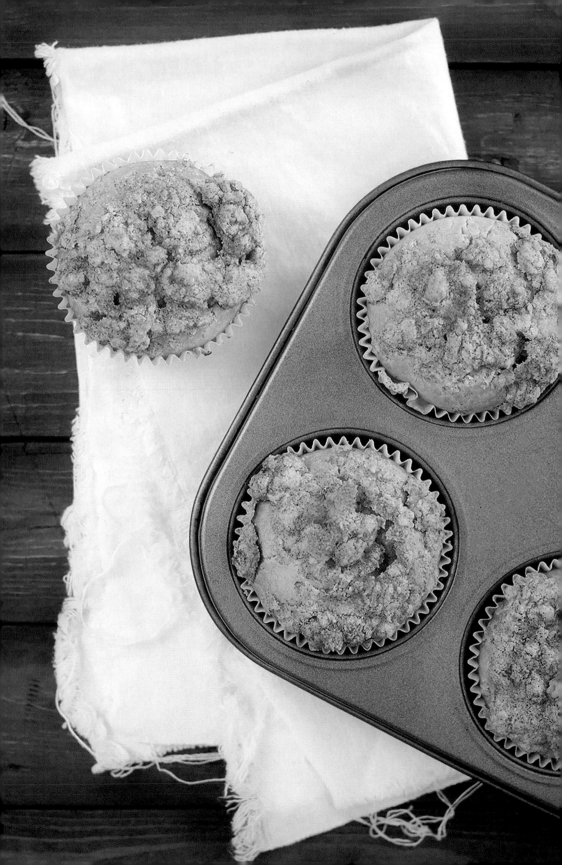

Sugar-free Cinnabites

Everybody loves a good cinnamon roll. Soft and warm on the inside, chewy on the outside — the perfect comfort food. With the same mouth-watering cinnamon taste, these sugar-free cinnabites make a fantastic substitute. They are great for finger food, breakfast, or a scrumptious dessert! Try topping them with a healthy cream cheese frosting for added indulgence.

Cake Batter

½ cup organic plain yogurt

¼ cup erythritol (like Swerve) or stevia, to taste

2 organic, pasture-raised eggs

2 ½ cups almond flour

¼ teaspoon Himalayan sea salt

½ teaspoon baking soda

Topping

2 tablespoons ground cinnamon

4 tablespoons erythritol (like Swerve), xylitol, or stevia, to taste

2 tablespoons organic unsalted butter or coconut butter, melted

Directions

Preheat oven to 310° F.

Combine all the wet ingredients for the batter into a bowl and blend well with a spoon. Add the dry ingredients for the batter and blend well with a spoon.

Blend all the topping ingredients using a fork.

Place cupcake liners in a muffin pan and fill the liners ⅔ with batter. Add small crumble of topping for mini muffins or about a tablespoon of topping for large muffins on top of the batter.

Use toothpick or skewer to mix some of the topping into the batter (or just leave it on top).

Bake for 20–25 minutes or until a toothpick placed in the center of a muffin comes out clean and the tops are starting to brown.

MAKES 12 CINNABITES

Almond Flour Lemon Bars

These lemon bars are a sugar-free, gluten-free, and paleo version of an old-fashioned favorite recipe that is great for any gathering. Use powdered xylitol to top off the smooth, custard filling and soft, chewy crust.

Crust

1 cup finely ground almond flour

¼ teaspoon Himalayan sea salt

2 tablespoons powdered xylitol

1 tablespoon coconut oil, melted

2 tablespoons raw unsalted organic butter, melted

1 tablespoon pure vanilla extract

Lemon Topping

¼ cup finely ground almond flour

¼ cup powdered xylitol

2 teaspoon stevia

4 large organic, pasture-raised eggs

½ cup fresh squeezed lemon juice

SERVES 4–6

Directions

Preheat oven to 350° F.

Line an 8-inch square baking dish with unbleached parchment paper.

Crust

Combine the almond flour, powdered xylitol, and sea salt in a large bowl. In a medium bowl, stir together coconut oil, butter, and vanilla extract.Stir the wet ingredients into the dry until thoroughly combined.

Press the dough evenly into the bottom of the prepared baking dish. Bake for 15 –17 minutes until lightly golden.

Lemon Topping

While the crust bakes, prepare the topping. In a blender or food processor (or by hand with a whisk), combine the almond flour, powdered xylitol, stevia, eggs, and lemon juice. Blend on medium speed until smooth.

Remove the crust from the oven. Pour the topping evenly over the hot crust. Pop back into oven. Bake for 15–20 minutes at 350° F until the topping is golden at edges.

Let cool in the baking dish for 30 minutes, then refrigerate for 2 hours to set.

Put ¼ cup xylitol in a coffee grinder until powdery with the same consistency of icing sugar. Sprinkle with powdered xylitol (optional).

Cut into bars and serve.

Whole Food Date Caramels

Did you know that when blended with coconut oil, dates make a healthy and delicious caramel-like filling? Make these whole food date caramels for the perfect salty-sweet dessert for your next party or event. Now you can enjoy one of your favorite flavors, free from refined sugar! **Inspired by Empowered Sustenance.**

1 packed cup pitted dates

¼ cup coconut milk (full fat or light), warmed

¼ cup melted coconut oil

½ teaspoon vanilla extract (optional)

¼ – ½ teaspoon Himalayan sea salt

Coconut flour, for dusting

Chocolate Coating

¼ cup cocoa powder

¼ cup coconut oil

Stevia, to taste

MAKES ABOUT 15 LARGE OR 25 SMALL CARAMELS

Directions

Soak dates in very hot water for 15 minutes. Drain before proceeding.

Blend the dates, coconut milk, coconut oil, and vanilla extract until a smooth paste forms. Add ¼ teaspoon salt, blend, and taste. Add a bit more salt if desired.

Place in the fridge or freezer until firm and pliable, at least 3 hours.

Roll teaspoons of the date mixture into balls. Dust lightly with coconut flour so they don't stick to each other. Place in the freezer to stay firm.

Melt and stir together the cocoa powder, coconut oil, and stevia over very low heat until combined. Let the mixture cool until thickened enough to coat the caramel balls.

Place in the fridge for a few minutes if it is too runny, but keep an eye on it because it hardens very quickly.

One by one, roll a caramel into the chocolate and place on a baking sheet lined with unbleached parchment or waxed paper. Sprinkle very lightly with the unrefined salt, and place in the fridge until the chocolate coating is firm.

Store in the fridge. If they aren't consumed quickly, they last at least a few weeks in the fridge.

Grain-free Chocolate Cupcakes

Cure your sweet tooth and fulfill chocolate cravings with this grain-free and sugar-free version of a classic dessert. You can also make these dairy-free by using coconut oil in the place of butter. Enjoy them as a snack or dessert by themselves, topped with frosting, chocolate ganache, or whipped cream, or served with a side of ice cream or strawberry gelato.

Cupcakes

2 cups pecans

1/3 cup unsweetened cocoa powder

1 teaspoon baking powder

¼ teaspoon Himalayan sea salt

4 organic, pasture-raised eggs

½ cup melted organic butter or coconut oil

1 teaspoon pure vanilla extract (sugar-free — check the label)

¼ teaspoon stevia extract powder

½ cup water, unsweetened almond milk, or coffee

Buttercream Frosting

1 cup organic butter

4 oz stevia sweetened chocolate chips (no sugar)

MAKES 10–12 CUPCAKES

Directions

Crust

Heat oven to 350° F. Line a muffin tin with silicone cups or paper liners.

Process pecans in food processor — pulse until they are meal, not quite as small as corn meal.

Add the rest of the dry ingredients and pulse again.

Add the wet ingredients and process until well-blended.

Separate into muffin cups (or small ramekins) and bake for 20–25 minutes.

> **NOTE** The exact time will vary with the pan. Start checking at 20 minutes. When toothpick inserted in center comes out clean, the cupcakes are done.

Lemon Topping

Gently melt together in a saucepan.

Pour the melted mixture into a bowl; chill for 2-3 hours.

With a hand-held mixer, beat the chilled mixture until it is light, fluffy, and spreadable. Apply on cupcakes.

Optional toppings

Chocolate ganache (See *Chocolate Truffles* on page 302)

Whipped cream

Primal Pots de Crème

Instead of serving pie, try this decadent, sugar-free, chocolate dessert — Primal Pots de Crème. It's a great option for anyone with dairy and nut- or grain-based allergies. Best of all, the preparation is easy! **Inspired by Elana's Pantry.**

1 can (13.5 ounces) coconut milk

2 organic, pasture-raised egg yolks

¼ teaspoon vanilla stevia

Pinch Himalayan sea salt

½ cup stevia sweetened organic chocolate chunks or chips

Directions

Place coconut milk in a medium saucepan. Stir in egg yolks, stevia, and salt. Heat over medium-heat 5–10 minutes, stirring constantly.

Remove saucepan from heat. Transfer mixture to blender or Vitamix® and add chocolate. Blend on high for 30 seconds.

Transfer ½ cup of mixture into 4 ramekins. Refrigerate overnight or for 8 hours. Serve.

SERVES 4

Raw Brownie Balls

Meet the solution to your next chocolate craving and cut out refined carbs and sugar with these raw brownie balls. The combination of dates, walnuts, and cocoa powder make these easy-to-make treats far more decadent than you'd expect.

1 cup walnuts or peanuts

6–10 pitted dates, soaked in water

½ teaspoon stevia, or to taste

1 cup unsweetened cocoa powder

2 teaspoons ghee or coconut oil

⅛ – ¼ cup shredded coconut, unsweetened

Directions

Put everything in the blender and mix.

Shape into one inch balls and refrigerate.

Serve cool or chilled.

MAKES 12–24 BALLS

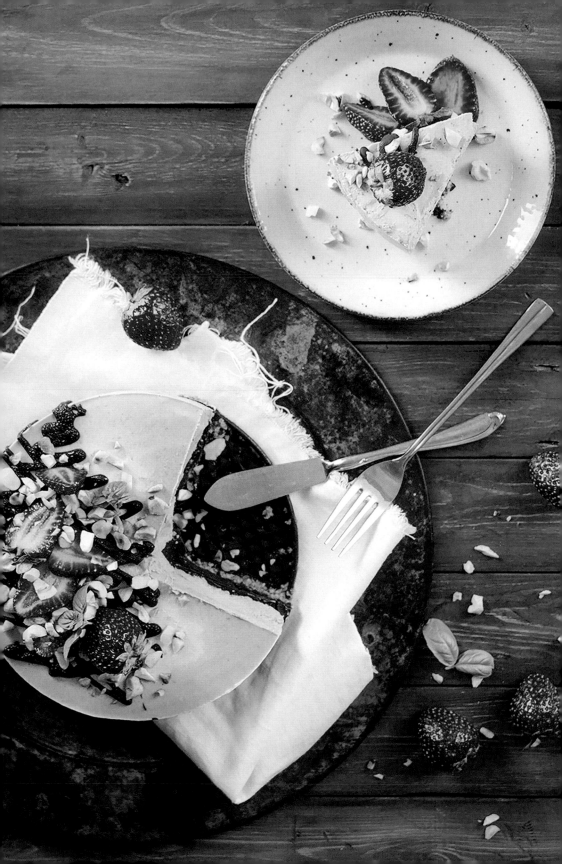

Black-Bottom Strawberry Pie

This no-bake pie will become your family's new favorite dessert. If you prefer a different flavor, substitute the fresh strawberries with raspberries or blueberries, or a combination. Most importantly, it's sugar-free, so you can indulge in a guilt-free dessert!

Crust

¾ cup crushed raw pecans or walnuts

¼ cup dried unsweetened shredded coconut

¾ cup stevia-sweetened* organic melted chocolate (optional)

Filling

2 cups fresh strawberries (or raspberries)

1 cup raw organic cashews

2 teaspoons vanilla extract (do not add if using liquid vanilla stevia)

1–2 droppers full of liquid stevia (to taste), or ⅛ – ¼ teaspoon pure stevia extract powder

1 pinch Himalayan sea salt

1 cup coconut oil, melted

Directions

Grind crust ingredients in food processor or high speed blender, and then press mixture into bottom of a 9-inch pie plate, building up the sides slightly.

If adding the "black bottom," pour the melted chocolate over the crust and cool in the fridge while you prepare the creamy strawberry filling.

Place all filling ingredients into blender or food processor to blend until smooth and creamy.

Carefully pour blended filling on top of crust and refrigerate for 2–3 hours.

MAKES 1 PIE

> *** NOTE** To sweeten melting chocolate, use approximately ⅛ of a teaspoon of powdered concentrated stevia. Liquid stevia may seize melting chocolate.

Cinnamon Spice Pecans

These are great to leave out as a sugar-free treat when company is over!

1 organic, pasture-raised egg white

10 drops of liquid stevia (vanilla flavor or original)

1 teaspoon Himalayan sea salt

1 teaspoon ground cinnamon

1 pinch of chipotle powder

2 cups pecans

Directions

In a large bowl, whisk together egg white, stevia, salt, chipotle and cinnamon. Toss nuts in the egg white mixture to coat. Pour nut mixture onto a parchment paper lined baking sheet. Bake at 300° for 15-20 minutes, until nuts are browned. Allow nuts to cool for 5 minutes, then break apart and serve

SERVES 6-8

Vegan Vanilla Ice Cream

With only four ingredients, you can quickly make this vegan ice cream to enjoy on a hot day or after dinner without feeling guilty. Serve it with your favorite dessert.

2 cups coconut water

1 cup raw cashews

1 tablespoon vanilla extract

10 drops liquid stevia

SERVES 2-4

Directions

Blend in Blendtec® or other high speed blender.

Add into ice cream maker, and enjoy.

Optional toppings

Organic strawberries, blueberries, raspberries, or mix of berries of your choice; chopped almonds, walnuts, or nuts of your choice; shredded unsweetened coconut flakes; raw cacao powder; cinnamon

Almond Butter Cups

These sugar-free treats will satisfy any chocolate cup connoisseur.
For a nut-free version, try substituting the almond butter for sunflower seed butter.

Chocolate

¼ cup organic butter
or coconut oil

3–4 squares unsweetened
organic chocolate

¼ teaspoon stevia
extract powder (may
adjust to taste)

Dash of cinnamon
(optional)

Almond Butter Filling

1 scoop vanilla plant-
based or organic grass-fed
whey protein powder

½ teaspoon
Himalayan sea salt

½ cup raw almond butter

1 tablespoon pure
vanilla (sugar-free —
check the label)

¼ cup organic butter
or coconut oil (or
a combination),
well softened

Directions

In a saucepan, melt butter/coconut oil and chocolate squares over very low heat. Remove from heat.

Add stevia, salt, and cinnamon to chocolate mixture.

Combine all the almond butter filling ingredients into a thick pudding by mashing with a fork. This takes some mixing, and is easier if your almond butter and butter/coconut oil are at room temperature.

Pour enough chocolate mixture to cover the very bottom of the cupcake papers. Use silicone muffin cups or a silpat mini muffin tin without any liner. If you do not have this, or cannot find one, use a regular or mini cupcake tin lined with regular or mini cupcake papers.

Use a small ice cream scoop or large melon baller to spoon a little of the almond butter filling on top of the chocolate coating.

Cover with the remaining chocolate mixture.

Chill to set.

Store in the refrigerator or the freezer.

MAKES ABOUT 12 CUPS

Chocolate Truffles

*These chocolate truffles complement your desserts without sugar and white flour.
This sweet treat can also be used as a frosting for chocolate cupcakes.*

8 oz. unsweetened organic baker's chocolate, chopped into tiny pieces

1 cup organic heavy cream

1 teaspoon pure vanilla (sugar-free — check the ingredients)

¼ teaspoon Himalayan sea salt

½ teaspoon stevia extract powder

1 teaspoon instant espresso powder (optional)

Directions

Heat the cream, vanilla, stevia, espresso powder, and salt until bubbles form. Remove from heat. Add chocolate pieces and let melt, stirring occasionally. Let the mixture cool to room temperature, and then chill slightly in the refrigerator. Roll into truffles, which you can then roll into chopped raw nuts, unsweetened shredded coconut, or unsweetened cocoa powder.

Optional toppings

Chopped raw nuts of your choice; unsweetened shredded coconut; unsweetened cocoa powder

MAKES 24 TRUFFLES

Chocolate Chunk Brownies

Is your sweet tooth at it again? Satisfy it with these delicious guilt-free chocolate chunk brownies. using raw almond butter, cocoa powder, and unsweetened dark chocolate, these brownies are sure to be a hit.

2 cups raw almond butter, smooth unroasted

2 organic, pasture-raised eggs

¼ teaspoon stevia

1 tablespoon vanilla extract

½ cup cocoa powder

½ teaspoon Himalayan sea salt

1 teaspoon baking soda

½ cup unsweetened chocolate, preferably organic

Directions

In a large bowl, blend almond butter until smooth with a hand blender. Blend in eggs, then blend in stevia and vanilla. Blend in cocoa, salt, and baking soda. Chop unsweetened chocolate into chunks and fold into brownie batter. Grease a 9 × 13 inch pyrex baking dish. Pour batter into dish. Bake at 325° F for 35–40 minutes. Store chilled.

MAKES 12 BROWNIES

References

Chapter 1

Chronic Disease Prevention and Health Promotion. (2017, June 28). Retrieved December 17, 2017, from https://www.cdc.gov/chronicdisease/overview/index.htm#ref17

Kanavos, et al. (2013, April). Higher US Branded Drug Prices And Spending Compared To Other Countries May Stem Partly From Quick Uptake Of New Drugs. Retrieved December 17, 2017, from https://www.healthaffairs.org/doi/abs/10.1377/hlthaff.2012.0920#

National Center for Health Statistics. (2017, May 03). Retrieved December 17, 2017, from https://www.cdc.gov/nchs/fastats/health-expenditures.htm

Twice As Many Moms Say They're Concerned About Their Weight Than That Of Their Children, But Grocery Purchases Are Driven by Health & Nutrition For Their Entire Family. (2014, May & june). Retrieved December 17, 2017, from http://www.womensforummediagroup.com/twice-as-many-moms-say-theyre-concerned-about-their-weight-than-that-of-their-children-but-grocery-purchases-are-driven-by-health-nutrition-for-their-entire-family/

Weinberg, S. L. (2004, March 03). The diet-heart hypothesis: a critique. Retrieved December 17, 2017, from https://www.ncbi.nlm.nih.gov/pubmed/14998608

Chapter 2

Bielecki, A., & Nieszporska, S. (2017). The proposal of philosophical basis of the health care system. Retrieved December 17, 2017, from https://www.ncbi.nlm.nih.gov/pmc/articles/PMC5318466/

Fos, P. J. (2011). *Epidemiology foundations the science of public health.* San Francisco, Ca.: Jossey-Bass.

Frequently asked questions. (n.d.). Retrieved December 17, 2017, from http://www.who.int/suggestions/faq/en/

Chapter 3

Brennan, P. C, et al. (1991, September). Enhanced phagocytic cell respiratory burst induced by spinal manipulation: potential role of substance P. Retrieved December 17, 2017, from https://www.ncbi.nlm.nih.gov/pubmed/1719112

Bryans, R, et al. (2011, June). Evidence-based guidelines for the chiropractic treatment of adults with headache. Retrieved December 17, 2017, from https://www.ncbi.nlm.nih.gov/pubmed/21640251

Chiropractic Paradigm / Scope & Practice. (n.d.). Retrieved December 19, 2017, from http://www.chirocolleges.org/resources/chiropractic-paradigm-scope-practice/

Hawk, C., DC. (2013, August 30). When Worldviews Collide: Maintaining a Vitalistic Perspective in Chiropractic in the Postmodern Era. Retrieved December 18, 2017, from http://www.sciencedirect.com/science/article/pii/S1556349913601473

Hightower, B. C., et al. (1994). THE EFFECTS OF SPECIFIC UPPER CERVICAL ADJUSTMENTS ON THE CD4 COUNTS OF HIV POSITIVE PATIENTS. Retrieved December 18, 2017, from https://www.chiroindex.org/?search_page=articles&action&articleId=5619

Keet , A. D., M.B. Ch. B. (n.d.). Chapter 8. *In The Pyloric Sphincteric Cylinder In Health and Disease.* Retrieved from http://med.plig.org/8/

Peterson, C. K., et al. (2014, April 01). Outcomes of pregnant patients with low back pain undergoing chiropractic treatment: a prospective cohort study with short term, medium term and 1 year follow-up. Retrieved December 18, 2017, from https://chiromt.biomedcentral.com/articles/10.1186/2045-709X-22-15

Teodorczyk-Injeyan, J. A., et al. (2010, September 08). Interleukin 2-regulated in vitro antibody production following a single spinal manipulative treatment in normal subjects. Retrieved December 17, 2017, from https://www.ncbi.nlm.nih.gov/pubmed/20825650

Torns, S. (2012). Retrieved December 17, 2017, from https://www.chiroindex.org/?search_page=articles&action&articleId=22580

University of Chicago Medical Center. "Special Chiropractic Adjustment Lowers Blood Pressure." ScienceDaily. ScienceDaily, 16 March 2007.

Vieira-Pellenz, F., et al. (2014, September). Short-term effect of spinal manipulation on pain perception, spinal mobility, and full height recovery in male subjects with degenerative disk disease: a randomized controlled trial. Retrieved December 18, 2017, from https://www.ncbi.nlm.nih.gov/pubmed/24862763

WFC Policy Statement. (n.d.). Retrieved https://www.wfc.org/website/docs/992003142614. PDF

Also see: Dr. Deed Harrison on idealspine.com and Dr. Heidi Haavik on chiropracticresearch.ac.nz

Chapter 4

Akther, F. (2016). Assessment of Nutritional Status & Health Condition Among Vegetarian and Non-vegetarian Adult at Tangail Sadar Upazila in Tangail District. *International Journal of Nutrition and Food Sciences,* 5(4), 241. doi:10.11648/j.ijnfs.20160504.12

Aquaculture. (n.d.). Retrieved December 20, 2017, from https://www.seafoodwatch.org/ocean-issues/aquaculture/pollution-and-disease

Bae, J., et al. (2012). Low Cholesterol is Associated with Mortality from Cardiovascular Diseases: A Dynamic Cohort Study in Korean Adults. *Journal of Korean Medical Science,* 27(1), 58. doi:10.3346/jkms.2012.27.1.58

Center for Food Safety and Applied Nutrition. (2017.). Food Additives & Ingredients - Everything Added to Food in the United States (EAFUS).

Center for Food Safety and Applied Nutrition. (2017.). Labeling & Nutrition - Guidance for Industry: Trans Fatty Acids in Nutrition Labeling, Nutrient Content Claims, Health Claims; Small Entity Compliance Guide.

Chang, C. Y., Ke, & Chen. (2009). Essential fatty acids and human brain. *Acta Neurologica Taiwanica ,* 18(4), 231-241. Retrieved from https://www.ncbi.nlm.nih.gov/pubmed/20329590.

Crosby, G. (2017, November 20). Ask the Expert: Concerns about canola oil. Retrieved December 20, 2017, from https://www.hsph.harvard.edu/nutritionsource/2015/04/13/ask-the-expert-concerns-about-canola-oil/

Davis, W., MD. (2012, January). A Wheat Farmer Weighs in on Wheat Belly [Web log post]. Retrieved from http://www.wheatbellyblog.com/2012/01/a-wheat-farmer-weighs-in-on-wheat-belly/

Darbre, P. D. (2017). Endocrine Disruptors and Obesity. Current Obesity Reports, 6(1), 18-27. doi:10.1007/s13679-017-0240-4

Elswyk, M. E., & Mcneill, S. H. (2014). Impact of grass/forage feeding versus grain finishing on beef nutrients and sensory quality: The U.S. experience. *Meat Science,* 96(1), 535-540. doi:10.1016/j.meatsci.2013.08.010

References

Fan , S. (2013, October 1). The fat-fueled brain: unnatural or advantageous? [Web log post]. Retrieved from https://blogs.scientificamerican.com/mind-guest-blog/the-fat-fueled-brain-unnatural-or-advantageous/

Food: Field to Fork. (n.d.). Retrieved December 20, 2017, from http://www.panna.org/food-farming-derailed/food-field-fork

Ford, E. S., & Capewell, S. (2007). Coronary Heart Disease Mortality Among Young Adults in the U.S. From 1980 Through 2002. *Journal of the American College of Cardiology, 50*(22), 2128-2132. doi:10.1016/j.jacc.2007.05.056

Grootveld, M., et al. (2001). Health Effects Of Oxidized Heated Oils[1]. *Foodservice Research International*, 13(1), 41-55. doi:10.1111/j.1745-4506.2001.tb00028.x

He, F., & Chen, J. (2013). Consumption of soybean, soy foods, soy isoflavones and breast cancer incidence: Differences between Chinese women and women in Western countries and possible mechanisms. F*ood Science and Human Wellness, 2*(3-4), 146-161. doi:10.1016/j.fshw.2013.08.002

Healthy Cooking Oils. (n.d.). Retrieved December 20, 2017, from https://recipes.heart.org/Articles/1013/Healthy-Cooking-Oils

Healthy Schools. (2017, January 25). Retrieved December 20, 2017, from https://www.cdc.gov/healthyschools/obesity/facts.htm

Heiden, M. G., Cantley, L. C., & Thompson, C. B. (2009). Understanding the Warburg Effect: The Metabolic Requirements of Cell Proliferation. *Science, 324*(5930), 1029-1033. doi:10.1126/science.1160809

How a Day's Worth of Sugary Drinks Adds Up to a whopping 93 Sugar Packets. (2014). *Queens Community Board 13 Newsletter* . Retrieved from http://www.nyc.gov/html/qnscb13/downloads/pdf/CB13Q_NEWSLETTER_0214.pdf

Kearns, C. E., Schmidt, L. A., & Glantz, S. A. (2016). Sugar Industry and Coronary Heart Disease Research. *JAMA Internal Medicine, 176*(11), 1680. doi:10.1001/jamainternmed.2016.5394

Liberti, M. V., & Locasale, J. W. (2016). The Warburg Effect: How Does it Benefit Cancer Cells? *Trends in Biochemical Sciences, 41*(3), 211-218. doi:10.1016/j.tibs.2015.12.001

Macpherson-Sánchez, A. E. (2015). Integrating Fundamental Concepts of Obesity and Eating Disorders: Implications for the Obesity Epidemic. *American Journal of Public Health, 105*(4). doi:10.2105/ajph.2014.302507

National Center for Health Statistics. (2017, March 17). Retrieved December 20, 2017, from https://www.cdc.gov/nchs/fastats/leading-causes-of-death.htm

Nöthlings, U., et al. (2005, October 05). Meat and fat intake as risk factors for pancreatic cancer: the multiethnic cohort study. Retrieved December 20, 2017, from https://www.ncbi.nlm.nih.gov/pubmed/16204695

Overweight & Obesity. (2017, August 29). Retrieved December 20, 2017, from https://www.cdc.gov/obesity/data/adult.html

Prediabetes & Insulin Resistance. (2009, August 01). Retrieved December 20, 2017, from https://www.niddk.nih.gov/health-information/diabetes/overview/what-is-diabetes/prediabetes-insulin-resistance

Ravnskov, U., et al. (2016). Lack of an association or an inverse association between low-density-lipoprotein cholesterol and mortality in the elderly: a systematic review. *BMJ Open, 6*(6). doi:10.1136/bmjopen-2015-010401

Red Meat. (n.d.). Retrieved from http://research.omicsgroup.org/index.php/Red_meat

Retrieved December 20, 2017, from http://www.betacasein.org/index.php?p=variants

Robbins, J. (2006). *Healthy at 100: The Scientifically Proven Secrets of the Worlds Healthiest and Longest-lived Peoples.* Thorndike/Windsor/Paragon.

Roizen, M. (2009). The Content of Favorable and Unfavorable Polyunsaturated Fatty Acids Found in Commonly Eaten Fish. *Yearbook of Anesthesiology and Pain Management, 2009,* 324-325. doi:10.1016/s1073-5437(09)79198-3

Sacks, F. M., et al (2017). Dietary Fats and Cardiovascular Disease. A Presidential Advisory From the American Heart Association. *Circulation, 136*(3) doi:10.1161/cir.0000000000000510

Samsel, A., & Seneff, S. (2013). Glyphosate's Suppression of Cytochrome P450 Enzymes and Amino Acid Biosynthesis by the Gut Microbiome: Pathways to Modern Diseases. *Entropy,15*(4), 1416-1463. doi:10.3390/e15041416

Scientific Report of the 2015 Dietary Advisory Committee [PDF]. (2015). USDA.

Silent Spring. (n.d.). Retrieved December 20, 2017, from http://www.encyclopedia.com/history/united-states-and-canada/us-history/silent-spring#3400500302

Trans fats, but not saturated fats like butter, linked to greater risk of early death and heart disease. (August 11, 2015.). *Science Daily.* Retrieved December 12, 2017.

What is Metabolic Syndrome [PDF]. (2015). American Heart Association.

World Health Organization Says Processed Meat Causes Cancer. (n.d.). Retrieved December 20, 2017, from https://www.cancer.org/latest-news/world-health-organization-says-processed-meat-causes-cancer.html

Chapter 5

Aragon, A., & Schoenfeld, B. (2013). Nutrient Timing Revisited. *Functional Foods*, 65–89. doi:10.1201/b16307-5

Brito, L. B., et al. (2014, July). Ability to sit and rise from the floor as a predictor of all-cause mortality. Retrieved December 18, 2017, from https://www.ncbi.nlm.nih.gov/pubmed/23242910

Diaz, K. M., et al. (2017, October 03). Patterns of Sedentary Behavior and Mortality in U.S. Middle-Aged and Older Adults: A National Cohort Study. Retrieved December 18, 2017, from http://annals.org/aim/article-abstract/2653704/patterns-sedentary-behavior-mortality-u-s-middle-aged-older-adults

Faris, M. A., et al. (2012, December). Intermittent fasting during Ramadan attenuates proinflammatory cytokines and immune cells in healthy subjects. Retrieved December 18, 2017, from https://www.ncbi.nlm.nih.gov/pubmed/23244540

Ho, K. Y., et al. (1988). Fasting enhances growth hormone secretion and amplifies the complex rhythms of growth hormone secretion in man. *Journal of Clinical Investigation*, *81*(4), 968–975. doi:10.1172/jci113450

Kemmler, W., et al. (2015, January). [High versus moderate intense running exercise - effects on cardiometabolic risk-factors in untrained males]. Retrieved December 18, 2017, from https://www.ncbi.nlm.nih.gov/pubmed/25580979

Klempel, M. C., et al. (2012). Intermittent fasting combined with calorie restriction is effective for weight loss and cardio-protection in obese women. *Nutrition Journal*, *11*(1). doi:10.1186/1475-2891-11-98

Levine, J., M.D., Ph.D. (2015, September 04). Too much sitting is bad for your health. Retrieved December 18, 2017, from https://www.mayoclinic.org/healthy-lifestyle/adult-health/expert-answers/sitting/faq-20058005

Loon, L. J., et al. (2003). Intramyocellular lipids form an important substrate source during moderate intensity exercise in endurance-trained males in a fasted state. *The Journal of Physiology*, *553*(2), 611–625. doi:10.1113/jphysiol.2003.052431

Mandal, A. C. (1986). The ergonomics of library issue desks. *Applied Ergonomics*, *17*(2), 140–141. doi:10.1016/0003-6870(86)90278-4

O'Riordan , M. (2012, June 6). The Not-So-Long Run: Mortality Benefit of Running Less Than 20 Miles per Week. Retrieved December 22, 2017, from https://www.medscape.com/viewarticle/765209

Pendergast, D., EdD. FACN. (2013, June). A Perspective on Fat Intake in Athletes. Retrieved December 18, 2017, from http://www.tandfonline.com/doi/abs/10.1080/07315724.2000.10718930?journalCode=uacn20&

Tipton, C. M. (2008). Susruta of India, an unrecognized contributor to the history of exercise physiology. *Journal of Applied Physiology, 104*(6), 1553-1556. doi:10.1152/japplphysiol.00925.2007

Varady, K. A., et al. (2009). Short-term modified alternate-day fasting: a novel dietary strategy for weight loss and cardioprotection in obese adults. *American Journal of Clinical Nutrition,90*(5), 1138-1143. doi:10.3945/ajcn.2009.28380

Chapter 6

5 Surprising Sources of Lead Exposure. (n.d.). Retrieved December 19, 2017, from https://www.webmd.com/children/lead#4

Bittner, G. D., Yang, C. Z., & Stoner, M. A. (2014). Estrogenic chemicals often leach from BPA-free plastic products that are replacements for BPA-containing polycarbonate products. *Environmental Health, 13*(1). doi:10.1186/1476-069x-13-41

Bøhn, T. (2014). Compositional differences in soybeans on the market: Glyphosate accumulates in Roundup Ready GM soybeans. *Food Chemistry, 153*, 207-215. doi:10.1016/j.foodchem.2013.12.054

Bouchard, M., et al. (2009). Blood Lead Levels and Major Depressive Disorder, Panic Disorder, and Generalized Anxiety Disorder in U.S. Young Adults. *Epidemiology, 20*. doi:10.1097/01.ede.0000362292.40972.3a

BPA and other Cord Blood Pollutants. Environmental Working Group. (2009, November 23). Retrieved December 19, 2017, from https://www.ewg.org/research/minority-cord-blood-report/bpa-and-other-cord-blood-pollutants#.Wjidn9-nFPZ

Braun, J. M., et al. (2013). Personal care product use and urinary phthalate metabolite and paraben concentrations during pregnancy among women from a fertility clinic. *Journal of Exposure Science and Environmental Epidemiology, 24*(5), 459-466. doi:10.1038/jes.2013.69

Ceniceros, S., & Brown, G. R. (1998). Acupuncture: A Review of Its History, Theories, and Indications. *Southern Medical Journal, 91*(12), 1121-1125. doi:10.1097/00007611-199812000-00005

References

Claudio, L. (2011). Planting Healthier Indoor Air. *Environmental Health Perspectives, 119*(10). doi:10.1289/ehp.119-a426

Cleaning Supplies and Your Health. (n.d.). Retrieved December 19, 2017, from https://www.ewg.org/guides/cleaners/content/cleaners_and_health#.WjlZV9-nFPZ

Cooper, G. S., Miller, F. W., & Germolec, D. R. (2002). Occupational exposures and autoimmune diseases. *International Immunopharmacology, 2*(2-3), 303-313. doi:10.1016/s1567-5769(01)00181-3

Hodges, R. E., & Minich, D. M. (2015). Modulation of Metabolic Detoxification Pathways Using Foods and Food-Derived Components: A Scientific Review with Clinical Application. *Journal of Nutrition and Metabolism, 2015,* 1-23. doi:10.1155/2015/760689

Harley, K. G., et al. (2016). Reducing Phthalate, Paraben, and Phenol Exposure from Personal Care Products in Adolescent Girls: Findings from the HERMOSA Intervention Study. *Environmental Health Perspectives, 124*(10). doi:10.1289/ehp.1510514

How does poor indoor air quality affect me or my child? (n.d.). Retrieved December 19, 2017, from https://iaq.zendesk.com/hc/en-us/articles/212107247-How-does-poor-indoor-air-quality-affect-me-or-my-child-

Järup, L. (2003). Hazards of heavy metal contamination. Retrieved December 18, 2017, from https://www.ncbi.nlm.nih.gov/pubmed/14757716

Jedrychowski, W., et al. (2006). Effects of Prenatal Exposure to Mercury on Cognitive and Psychomotor Function in One-Year-Old Infants: Epidemiologic Cohort Study in Poland. *Annals of Epidemiology, 16*(6), 439-447. doi:10.1016/j.annepidem.2005.06.059

Known and Probable Human Carcinogens. (n.d.). Retrieved December 18, 2017, from https://www.cancer.org/cancer/cancer-causes/general-info/known-and-probable-human-carcinogens.html

Kumar, et al. (2012). Harmful effects of pesticides on human health. Annals of Agri Bio Research. 17. 165-168.

Maurya, S. (2015). Śodhana: An Ayurvedic process for detoxification and modification of therapeutic activities of poisonous medicinal plants. *Ancient Science of Life, 34*(4), 188. doi:10.4103/0257-7941.160862

McCauley, L. A., et al. (2006, June). Studying Health Outcomes in Farmworker Populations Exposed to Pesticides. Retrieved December 19, 2017, from https://www.ncbi.nlm.nih.gov/pmc/articles/PMC1480483/

Merrill, M., et al. (2012). Toxicological Function of Adipose Tissue: Focus on Persistent Organic Pollutants. Environmental Health Perspectives, 121(2), 162-169. doi:10.1289/ehp.1205485

Mitro, S. D., et al. (2016). Correction to Consumer Product Chemicals in Indoor Dust: A Quantitative Meta-Analysis of U.S. Studies. *Environmental Science & Technology, 50*(24), 13611-13611. doi:10.1021/acs.est.6b05530

National Primary Drinking Water Regulations. (2017, July 11). Retrieved December 19, 2017, from https://www.epa.gov/ground-water-and-drinking-water/national-primary-drinking-water-regulations

Peshin, S. S., Lall, S. B., & Gupta, S. K. (2002, March). Potential food contaminants and associated health risks. Retrieved December 19, 2017, from https://www.ncbi.nlm.nih.gov/pubmed/11918841

Pieper, K. J., et al. (2015). Incidence of waterborne lead in private drinking water systems in Virginia. *Journal of Water and Health, 13*(3), 897-908. doi:10.2166/wh.2015.275

Risk Management for Per- and Polyfluoroalkyl Substances (PFASs) under TSCA. (2017, December 13). Retrieved December 19, 2017, from https://www.epa.gov/assessing-and-managing-chemicals-under-tsca/risk-management-and-polyfluoroalkyl-substances-pfass

Smith, R. L. (2011). Slow Death by Rubber Duck: the Secret Danger of Everyday Things. Pgw.

UNITED STATES DEPARTMENT OF LABOR. (n.d.). Retrieved December 19, 2017, from https://www.osha.gov/SLTC/molds/hazards.html

Wijesekara, G., et al. (2015). Environmental and occupational exposures as a cause of male infertility: A caveat. *Ceylon Medical Journal, 60*(2), 52. doi:10.4038/cmj.v60i2.7090

Winter, C. K. (2012, February 15). Pesticide Residues in Imported, Organic, and. Retrieved December 19, 2017, from http://pubs.acs.org/doi/abs/10.1021/jf205131q

Yang, S. (2014, November). The Effects of Environmental Toxins on Allergic Inflammation. Retrieved December 18, 2017, from https://www.ncbi.nlm.nih.gov/pmc/articles/PMC4214967/

Chapter 7

Activated Charcoal (By mouth) - National Library of Medicine - PubMed Health. (n.d.). Retrieved December 19, 2017, from https://www.ncbi.nlm.nih.gov/pubmedhealth/PMHT0008816/?report=details

Adams, Ingrid. 2013. The Health Benefits of Dark Green Leafy Vegetables. Retrieved December 19, 2017 from http://www2.ca.uky.edu/agcomm/pubs/fcs3/fcs3567/fcs3567.pdf

Antioxidants: In Depth. (2016, May 04). Retrieved December 19, 2017, from https://nccih.nih.gov/health/antioxidants/introduction.htm

Babault, N. (2015). Pea proteins oral supplementation promotes muscle thickness gains during resistance training: a double-blind, randomized, Placebo-controlled clinical trial vs. Whey protein. *Journal of the International Society of Sports Nutrition, 12*(1), 3. doi:10.1186/s12970-014-0064-5

Bartnikowska , E., et al. (1997). [Unsaturated fatty acids omega-3. I. Structure, sources, determination, metabolism in the organism]. *Rocz Panstw Zakl Hig, 48*(4), 381-397. Retrieved from https://www.ncbi.nlm.nih.gov/pubmed/9562807.

Bennett, D. C., et al. (2011). Effect of diatomaceous earth on parasite load, egg production, and egg quality of free-range organic laying hens. *Poultry Science, 90*(7), 1416-1426. doi:10.3382/ps.2010-01256

Bischoff-Ferrari, H. A., et al. (2009). Benefit–risk assessment of vitamin D supplementation. *Osteoporosis International, 21*(7), 1121–1132. doi:10.1007/s00198-009-1119-3

Bounous, G., et al (1989). The influence of dietary whey protein on tissue glutathione and the diseases of aging. *Médecine clinique et expérimentale, 12*(6), 343-349. Retrieved from https://www.ncbi.nlm.nih.gov/pubmed/2692897.

Brown, M. A., Stevenson, E. J., & Howatson, G. (2017). Whey protein hydrolysate supplementation accelerates recovery from exercise-induced muscle damage in females. *Applied Physiology, Nutrition, and Metabolism.* doi:10.1139/apnm-2017-0412

Butler, C. C. (2006). Oral vitamin B12 versus intramuscular vitamin B12 for vitamin B12 deficiency: a systematic review of randomized controlled trials. *Family Practice, 23*(3), 279-285. doi:10.1093/fampra/cml008

Cameron-Smith, D., Albert, B. B., & Cutfield, W. S. (2015). Fishing for answers: is oxidation of fish oil supplements a problem? *Journal of Nutritional Science, 4.* doi:10.1017/jns.2015.26

Davis, D., PhD, Epp, M., PhD, & Riordan, H., MD. (1999). *Changes in USDA Food Composition Data for 43 Garden Crops, 1950 to 1999* [PDF]. Kansas City : Bio-Communications Research Institute.

Derlet , R., MD, & Albertson, T., MD, PhD. (1986). Activated Charcoal—Past, Present and Future. *Western Journal of Medicine, 145*(4), 493-496. Retrieved from https://www.ncbi.nlm.nih.gov/pmc/articles/PMC1306980/?page=4.

Elokda, A. S., & Nielsen, D. H. (2007). Effects of exercise training on the glutathione antioxidant system. *European Journal of Cardiovascular Prevention & Rehabilitation, 14*(5), 630-637. doi:10.1097/hjr.0b013e32828622d7

Farrah, S. R., et al. (1991, September 01). S R Farrah. Retrieved December 19, 2017, from http://aem.asm.org/content/57/9/2502

Fields, H. (2015, November). The Gut: Where Bacteria and Immune System Meet. Retrieved December 19, 2017, from https://www.hopkinsmedicine.org/research/advancements-in-research/fundamentals/in-depth/the-gut-where-bacteria-and-immune-system-meet

Hosseini, S. A., et al. (2014). The insecticidal effect of diatomaceous earth against adults and nymphs of Blattella germanica. *Asian Pacific Journal of Tropical Biomedicine, 4*. doi:10.12980/apjtb.4.2014c1282

Ismail, Y., Ismail, A. A., & Ismail, A. A. (2010). The underestimated problem of using serum magnesium measurements to exclude magnesium deficiency in adults; a health warning is needed for "normal" results. *Clinical Chemistry and Laboratory Medicine, 48*(3). doi:10.1515/cclm.2010.077

Jahnen-Dechent, W., & Ketteler, M. (2012). Magnesium basics. *Clinical Kidney Journal, 5*(Suppl 1), I3-I14. doi:10.1093/ndtplus/sfr163

Jeewanthi, R. K., Lee, N., & Paik, H. (2015). Improved Functional Characteristics of Whey Protein Hydrolysates in Food Industry. *Korean Journal for Food Science of Animal Resources, 35*(3), 350-359. doi:10.5851/kosfa.2015.35.3.350

Joseph, M. A., et al. (2004). Cruciferous Vegetables, Genetic Polymorphisms in Glutathione S-Transferases M1 and T1, and Prostate Cancer Risk. *Nutrition and Cancer, 50*(2), 206-213. doi:10.1207/s15327914nc5002_11

Moosavi, M. (2017). Bentonite Clay as a Natural Remedy: A Brief Review. *Iranian Journal of Public Health, 46*(9), 1176-1183. Retrieved from https://www.ncbi.nlm.nih.gov/pmc/articles/PMC5632318/.

Langan, R. C., & Goodbred, A. J. (2017). Vitamin B12 Deficiency: Recognition and Management. *American Family Physician, 96*(6), 384-389. Retrieved from https://www.ncbi.nlm.nih.gov/pubmed/28925645.

Merget, R., et al. (2002). Health hazards due to the inhalation of amorphous silica. *Archives of Toxicology, 75*(11-12), 625-34. Retrieved from https://www.ncbi.nlm.nih.gov/pubmed/11876495.

Nair, R., & Maseeh, A. (2012). Vitamin D: The "sunshine" vitamin. Retrieved December 19, 2017, from https://www.ncbi.nlm.nih.gov/pmc/articles/PMC3356951/

Naeem, Z. (2010, January). Vitamin D Deficiency- An Ignored Epidemic. Retrieved December 19, 2017, from https://www.ncbi.nlm.nih.gov/pmc/articles/PMC3068797/

Office of Dietary Supplements - Multivitamin/mineral Supplements. (n.d.).
  Retrieved December 19, 2017, from https://ods.od.nih.gov/factsheets/MVMS-
  HealthProfessional/#en3

Office of Dietary Supplements - Vitamin D. (n.d.). Retrieved December 19, 2017, from
  https://ods.od.nih.gov/factsheets/VitaminD-HealthProfessional/

Patrick , L., ND. (2002). Mercury Toxicity and Antioxidants: Part I: Role of Glutathione and
  alpha-Lipoic Acid in the Treatment of Mercury Toxicity. *Alternative Medicine Review* ,
  7(6), 456-471. Retrieved from http://www.altmedrev.com/publications/7/6/456.pdf

Richie , J. P., Jr., et al. (2014). Randomized controlled trial of oral glutathione
  supplementation on body stores of glutathione. *European Journal of Nutrition*, 54(2), 251-
  263. doi:10.1007/s00394-014-0706-z

Rock, C. L. (2007, January). Multivitamin-multimineral supplements: who uses
  them? Retrieved December 19, 2017, from https://www.ncbi.nlm.nih.gov/
  pubmed/17209209?dopt=Abstract

Rushton, L. (2007). Chronic Obstructive Pulmonary Disease and Occupational Exposure to
  Silica. *Reviews on Environmental Health*, 22(4). doi:10.1515/reveh.2007.22.4.255

Saini, R. (2011). Coenzyme Q10: The essential nutrient. *Journal of Pharmacy and Bioallied
  Sciences*, 3(3), 466. doi:10.4103/0975-7406.84471

Singh, N., et al. (2011). An Overview on Ashwagandha: A Rasayana (Rejuvenator) of
  Ayurveda. African Journal of Traditional, Complementary and Alternative Medicines,
  8(5S). doi:10.4314/ajtcam.v8i5s.9

Singh, V. P., et al. (2013, February). Role of probiotics in health and disease: A review.
  Retrieved December 19, 2017, from http://jpma.org.pk/full_article_text.php?article_
  id=4007

Silica-ItsNotJustDust [PDF]. (n.d.). UCONN.

Swanson, D., Block, R., & Mousa, S. A. (2012). Omega-3 Fatty Acids EPA and DHA: Health
  Benefits Throughout Life. *Advances in Nutrition: An International Review Journal*, 3(1), 1-7.
  doi:10.3945/an.111.000893

Test ID: MTHFR   5,10-Methylenetetrahydrofolate Reductase C677T, Mutation, Blood.
  (n.d.). Retrieved December 20, 2017, from https://www.mayomedicallaboratories.com/
  test-catalog/Clinical and Interpretive/81648

Wani, A. L., Bhat, S. A., & Ara, A. (2015). Omega-3 fatty acids and the treatment of
  depression: a review of scientific evidence. *Integrative Medicine Research*, 4(3), 132-141.
  doi:10.1016/j.imr.2015.07.003

Ward, E. (2014). Addressing nutritional gaps with multivitamin and mineral supplements. *Nutrition Journal, 13*(1). doi:10.1186/1475-2891-13-72

Wierzbicka, G., et al. (1989). Glutathione in food. *Journal of Food Composition and Analysis, 2*(4), 327-337. doi:10.1016/0889-1575(89)90004-5

Wirunsawanya, K., et al. (2017). Whey Protein Supplementation Improves Body Composition and Cardiovascular Risk Factors in Overweight and Obese Patients: A Systematic Review and Meta-Analysis. *Journal of the American College of Nutrition,* 1-11. doi:10.1080/07315724.2017.1344591

Chapter 8

Al-Abri, M. A., et al. (2016). Habitual Sleep Deprivation is Associated with Type 2 Diabetes: A Case-Control Study. *Oman Medical Journal, 31*(6), 399-403. doi:10.5001/omj.2016.81

Arredondo, M., et al. (2017). A mindfulness training program based on brief practices (M-PBI) to reduce stress in the workplace: a randomised controlled pilot study. *International Journal of Occupational and Environmental Health,* 1-12. doi:10.1080/1077352 5.2017.1386607

Bankar, M., Chaudhari, S., & Chaudhari, K. (2013). Impact of long term Yoga practice on sleep quality and quality of life in the elderly. *Journal of Ayurveda and Integrative Medicine, 4*(1), 28. doi:10.4103/0975-9476.109548

Bin, Y. S., Marshall, N. S., & Glozier, N. (2013). Sleeping at the Limits: The Changing Prevalence of Short and Long Sleep Durations in 10 Countries. *American Journal of Epidemiology, 177*(8), 826-833. doi:10.1093/ajc/kws308

Chennaoui, M., et al. (2015). Sleep and exercise: A reciprocal issue? *Sleep Medicine Reviews, 20,* 59-72. doi:10.1016/j.smrv.2014.06.008

Figueiro, M., & Overington, D. (2016). Self-luminous devices and melatonin suppression in adolescents. *Lighting Research & Technology, 48*(8), 966-975. doi:10.1177/1477153515584979

Goldberg, S. B., et al. (2018). Mindfulness-based interventions for psychiatric disorders: A systematic review and meta-analysis. *Clinical Psychology Review, 59,* 52-60. doi:10.1016/j.cpr.2017.10.011

Grandner, M. A., et al. (2013). Sleep symptoms associated with intake of specific dietary nutrients. *Journal of Sleep Research, 23*(1), 22-34. doi:10.1111/jsr.12084

Hayashi, K., et al. (2016). Laughter is the Best Medicine? A Cross-Sectional Study of Cardiovascular Disease Among Older Japanese Adults. *Journal of Epidemiology, 26*(10), 546-552. doi:10.2188/jea.je20150196

References

Hill, P. L., Allemand, M., & Roberts, B. W. (2013). Examining the pathways between gratitude and self-rated physical health across adulthood. *Personality and Individual Differences, 54*(1), 92-96. doi:10.1016/j.paid.2012.08.011

Liu, Y., et al. (2016). Prevalence of Healthy Sleep Duration among Adults — United States, 2014. *MMWR. Morbidity and Mortality Weekly Report, 65*(6), 137-141. doi:10.15585/mmwr.mm6506a1

Madhav, K., Sherchand, S. P., & Sherchan, S. (2017). Association between screen time and depression among US adults. *Preventive Medicine Reports, 8*, 67-71. doi:10.1016/j.pmedr.2017.08.005

Mah, L., Szabuniewicz, C., & Fiocco, A. J. (2016). Can anxiety damage the brain? *Current Opinion in Psychiatry, 29*(1), 56-63. doi:10.1097/yco.0000000000000223

Minkel, J., et al. (2014). Sleep deprivation potentiates HPA axis stress reactivity in healthy adults. *Health Psychology, 33*(11), 1430-1434. doi:10.1037/a0034219

Pires, G. N., et al. (2016). Effects of acute sleep deprivation on state anxiety levels: a systematic review and meta-analysis. *Sleep Medicine, 24*, 109-118. doi:10.1016/j.sleep.2016.07.019

Roberts, C. J., Campbell, I. C., & Troop, N. (2013). Increases in Weight during Chronic Stress are Partially Associated with a Switch in Food Choice towards Increased Carbohydrate and Saturated Fat Intake. *European Eating Disorders Review, 22*(1), 77-82. doi:10.1002/erv.2264

Shechter, A., et al. (2018). Blocking nocturnal blue light for insomnia: A randomized controlled trial. *Journal of Psychiatric Research, 96*, 196-202. doi:10.1016/j.jpsychires.2017.10.015

Williams, P. G., et al. (2013). The Effects of Poor Sleep on Cognitive, Affective, and Physiological Responses to a Laboratory Stressor. *Annals of Behavioral Medicine, 46*(1), 40-51. doi:10.1007/s12160-013-9482-x

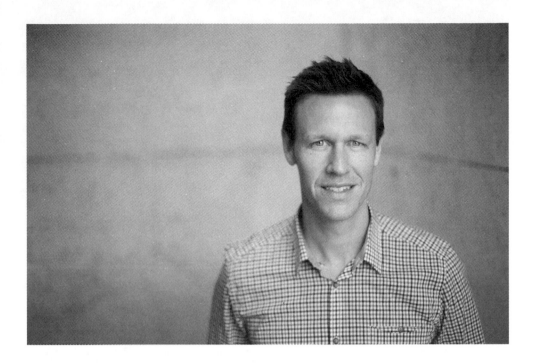

About the author

Dr. B.J. Hardick

Raised in a holistic family, Dr. B.J. Hardick is a Doctor of Chiropractic, organic foodie and fanatic for green living and earthly sustainability.

Dr. Hardick received his Bachelor of Science in Life Sciences from Queen's University in 1997, and his Doctorate of Chiropractic from Life University in 2001. He maintains a private practice in London, Ontario, Canada and has spent the majority of his life working in natural health care. In 2009, he authored his first book, *Maximized Living Nutrition Plans*. Today, he serves on the Board of Managers for MaxLiving, providing strategic guidance and inspiration. Dr. Hardick is committed to the advancement of holistic wellness education for chiropractors, health professionals, and anyone interested in achieving a balanced, healthy life.